Co

APPROACH

The CommonSense Approach Series

This series of self-help guides from Newleaf provides practical and sound ways to deal with many of life's common complaints.

Each book in the series is written for the layperson, and adopts a commonsense approach to the many questions surrounding a particular topic. It explains what the complaint is, how and why it occurs, and what can be done about it. It includes advice on helping ourselves, and information on where to go for further help. It encourages us to take responsibility for our own health, to be sensible and not always to rely on medical intervention for every ill.

AVAILABLE IN THIS SERIES

Addiction — The CommonSense Approach   Michael Hardiman

Menopause — The CommonSense Approach   Ruth Appleby

Stress — The CommonSense Approach   Brenda O'Hanlon

Sleep

THE

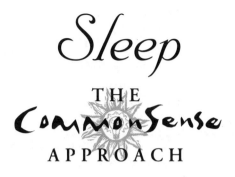

CommonSense

APPROACH

Brenda O'Hanlon

Newleaf

Newleaf

an imprint of
Gill & Macmillan Ltd
Hume Avenue, Park West
Dublin 12
with associated companies throughout the world
www.gillmacmillan.ie
© Brenda O'Hanlon 1998
0 7171 2628 5
This edition produced for Igloo Books Ltd,
Henson Way, Kettering, NN16 8PX.
info@igloo-books.com
Index compiled by Helen Litton
Design by Identikit Design Consultants, Dublin
Print origination by Carole Lynch
Printed in Malaysia

This book is typeset in Revivial565 9.5pt on 15pt.

A catalogue record for this book is available
from the British Library.

3 5 7 6 4

Contents

Foreword by Dr Chris Idzikowski   vii

Did You Know That ... ?   1

Chapter 1   4
All About Sleep

Chapter 2   11
How Much Sleep Do We Need?

Chapter 3   16
Common Sleep Disorders

Chapter 4   39
How to Get a Better Night's Sleep

Chapter 5   55
Getting Help

Chapter 6   68
Sleep Clinics

Chapter 7   74
Autogenic Training, Homeopathy and Acupuncture

Chapter 8   86
Complementary Medicine and Therapies
    Herbal Medicine
    Aromatherapy

Useful Addresses   104

Further Reading   108

Index   110

While the author has made every effort to ensure that the information contained in this book is accurate, it should not be regarded as an alternative to professional medical advice. Readers should consult their general practitioners or physicians if they are concerned about aspects of their own health, and before embarking on any course of treatment. Neither the author, nor the publishers, can accept responsibility for any health problem resulting from using, or discontinuing, any of the drugs described here, or the self-help methods described.

Foreword

Sleep is a fundamental state of being, yet the stresses of everyday life — illness, caring for others, a panoply of different factors — all can conspire to make it difficult. Everyone knows what it is like when sleep has been disturbed: inattention, irritability, tiredness and general malaise.

Research in the last thirty years has increased our knowledge concerning sleep, but little of this is percolating into a general awareness. Many healthcare professionals, including medical doctors, know little more than the general public. Therefore books like *Sleep: The CommonSense Approach* provide a tremendously useful bridge between contemporary knowledge and practical assistance.

Sleep in industrialised societies does not come naturally. The first one to two years of life are spent training babies to sleep according to the demands of our contemporary life styles. Sometimes this learning breaks down and 'disturbed' sleep results in later life. Life events such as bereavement, divorce and change of job can initially disturb sleep, but the disturbed sleep may not return to normal. The resultant chronic insomnia may be difficult to treat but might not have developed at all if remedial action had been taken straight away.

Societies generally do not tolerate individuals who cannot manage their mental state. Research shows that poor sleepers rarely achieve good jobs and often can develop disorders such as depression.

Recent research has shown that disturbed sleep costs the American economy at least 100 billion dollars a year through accidents, reduced productivity, absenteeism, hospitalisation, depression and alcoholism. Shift work is a necessary part of industrialised society, but inappropriate management of sleep can be more costly than ignoring it. Chernobyl, Three Mile

Island, the decision to launch Challenger, *Exxon Valdez*, various rail disasters, even the death of Princess Diana — all have involved sleep-disrupted individuals. Accidents should not be surprising, as there are virtually no good shift work rotas that take account of the biology of the brain's sleep wake systems. Doctors and nurses who have to work overnight are professional groups who also suffer from more accidents than those not involved in shift work.

Currently, many countries are reducing permissible alcohol levels in drivers. These levels are already below the equivalent performance impairment caused by a disrupted night's sleep.

Self-medication with alcohol is more likely to cause alcoholism than to improve sleep long-term. Melatonin is now popular in many countries but it is almost certainly abused as its effects on sleep and wakefulness are complex.

It is difficult to find anyone who has not had a disturbed night's sleep. For many this is a one-off event and sleep is restored the next or following night. As one gets older, though, sleep becomes more fragile and the various afflictions of old age take their toll. Sleeping pills are not necessarily the answer and may in some cases compound the problem. On the other hand, the individual may relearn to control their sleep if they are told what to do. Various research studies have shown that sleep education can improve the way people sleep and, unlike weight control, the improvement is maintained long-term.

Most measures of 'quality of life' assess sleep as an important variable. Everyone with disturbed sleep knows that it is. Yet the majority is ignorant of the facts. This book provides an excellent, thorough and practical approach to dealing with sleep problems.

Dr Chris Idzikowski

Director, Sleep Assessment and Advisory Service, Lisburn

Chairman, British Sleep Society, 1995–7

Founding Chairman, Royal Society of Medicine Forum on Sleep and its Disorders

Did You Know That ... ?

- Several studies have shown that hypnotics (the most commonly prescribed sleeping pills) are really only a short-term solution. To avoid habit formation, the maximum recommended use is for twenty-one days; even within that period, hypnotics are best taken on a non-consecutive basis.
- You always sleep worse when you stop taking sleeping pills, but this should only last a short time.
- A recent study shows that most sleep disorders specialists do not use sleeping pills to control their own short-term sleeping problems.
- The incidence of falls and hip fractures is higher among older people who are taking long-acting sleeping pills.
- Valerian is an alternative to sleeping pills for dealing with mild insomnia. It is widely available in pharmacies and health food stores.
- Between one-fifth and one-quarter of the adult population is affected by disturbed sleep in some form, and about one third by insomnia specifically. In psychiatric conditions, the figure is much higher.
- Sleeping problems are probably the second most frequently reported health problem, the common cold being the first.
- It has been found that the population at large takes at least a week to adjust to the effects of the summer/winter clock time change.
- Most people's sleep cycles are ninety minutes long. If you're taking a nap, it should only be for forty-five minutes, or at most ninety minutes.

◆ Sudden weight loss or gain can affect previously normal sleep patterns. Fragmented sleep may result from weight loss, whereas long and continuous sleep may result from weight gain.

◆ In the US, an estimated forty million people suffer from chronic sleep disorders and an unknown number have less severe sleeping problems. The cost to society is estimated at at least 100 billion dollars.

◆ One in five motorway accidents in Britain has been attributed to sleep disorders. In the US, sleep deprivation is reckoned to be the cause of 100,000 traffic accidents and 10,000 traffic fatalities each year.

◆ Chronic insomniacs have up to three times as many car accidents as good sleepers.

◆ Other studies show that one in five drivers admit to having fallen asleep at the wheel at least once.

◆ The rate of alcoholism among insomniacs is twice that of good sleepers.

◆ Insomnia is more common in adult women, especially those living alone and, as some studies show, also in the lower socio-economic groups. It is about equally likely in both men and women from their sixties onwards.

◆ Insomnia can be fatal. The rare illness, fatal familial insomnia, begins with difficulty falling asleep and soon leads to a total lack of sleep. It is always fatal within seven to thirteen months of onset.

◆ As we age, our sleep patterns change and our bodies become less adept at sustaining sleep at night. This may lead to taking more frequent naps during the day.

◆ One of the greatest myths of all is that alcohol helps sleep. You may fall asleep more quickly, but you'll wake up more often and earlier.

◆ Smoking before bed should also be avoided. Apart from all the other health reasons for not smoking, nicotine is a strong stimulant and may delay sleep onset. Research shows that the average smoker sleeps about thirty minutes less than a non-smoker.

- A high percentage of road traffic accidents occur around three in the afternoon and three in the morning. These times coincide with dips in our circadian rhythms and consequent periods of fatigue.

- During a normal night's sleep, we have four or five episodes of REM (dream) sleep. The first of these begins about ninety to 120 minutes after falling asleep. We tend to remember only those dreams that occurred immediately before waking.

- People with a normal sleep pattern wake up briefly every ninety minutes, but are usually unaware of it.

- Many sleeping pills depress both REM and deep sleep. The long-term side-effects of this are not known.

- Foetuses spend most of their time in REM sleep. New-born babies spend about half their time in REM sleep.

- Early morning awakening tends to be a symptom of depression. The sleep of depressed people is usually unrefreshing; they spend less time in Stage 3 and 4 (deep sleep).

- In the course of their training, medical students receive only about two hours' training in sleep disorders. Clinical psychologists receive only five minutes.

- The longest reported period of voluntary wakefulness was achieved by a seventeen-year-old Californian student. He was taking part in a sleep study experiment, and managed to stay awake for eleven days. After that, he slept for only fifteen hours, and apparently suffered no other side-effects.

- Day sleep after night work is, on average, two to four hours shorter than night sleep.

- Insomnia can be a symptom as well as a cause of general difficulties. Like a fever, it suggests that something is amiss, but in itself does not indicate what the problem is.

CHAPTER 1

All About Sleep

Some Historical Background

Once upon a time — well, for thousands and thousands of years actually — we all more or less worked from sunrise to sunset, returned home at twilight and, as night descended, went to bed. And from there to sleep. That night's sleep normally totalled somewhere between nine and ten hours. Then, suddenly, in 1879, along came the light bulb inventor and famous insomniac, Thomas Edison. As a direct result of his invention, people's activities and work were no longer constrained by lack of light and so they were obliged, or they chose, to devote more time to work or leisure activities. From around that time, our sleep patterns started to go out of sync.

One manifestation of just how out of sync they now are is the phenomenal sales of sleeping tablets world wide. For example, in the UK in 1992 (the latest year for which figures are available) doctors wrote twelve million prescriptions for hypnotics (sleeping pills). In the period 1980 to 1992, prescription figures declined only a little, from a high of 13.6 million. In that same twelve-year period, benzodiazepine (tranquilliser) prescriptions dropped dramatically from 18.9 million to 8.6 million. Why consumption figures for sleeping pills have remained so high against a background of almost continuous negative publicity is very puzzling indeed.

These days, the average urbanised Westerner is probably sleeping only six to eight hours a night. What is particularly significant about this is the speed of this change — nothing for tens of thousands of years, then a drop of over one-fifth in the last fifty years or so. In evolutionary terms, it's the equivalent of the blink of an eye.

Overall, we're not doing well in the sleep stakes — some worse than others, depending on their overall health, work, lifestyle, family circumstances or other pressures. Most experts agree that sleeping problems have now assumed epidemic proportions.

Sometimes the manifestations of sleep deprivation and trying to stay awake contrary to body-clock time can be disastrous. A number of researchers believe that this type of situation may have contributed to some of the most catastrophic industrial accidents of recent times. These include the poison gas leak at the Bhopal chemical plant in India; the explosion of the Challenger space shuttle; the Chernobyl nuclear power plant meltdown; and the near meltdown at the Three Mile Island nuclear power plant in the US. At a more routine level, sleep — or the lack of it — is blamed for tens of thousands of traffic accidents in the US each year. Nodding off for a few seconds (microsleep) can be fatal.

Is Sleep Necessary?

Why can't we stay awake all the time? Why should we spend one-third of our lives in a comatose condition? Why can't we imitate the seventeen-year-old Californian student who, in a specially designed experiment, survived eleven sleepless days and nights without any apparent ill effects?

The quick answer is that sleep architecture and the workings of the brain are extremely complex and require very careful synchronisation to work properly. So simple answers do not apply.

To understand sleep, you need to have some appreciation of the scientific process that goes on while you are asleep.

What the Experts Say

Dr Catherine Crowe is a sleep disorders specialist. A member of the European Sleep Research Society, she qualified as a psychiatrist before continuing her training at the Stanford University Sleep Disorders Laboratory in California. Later, she worked in France for several years. She now runs one of the few multi-disciplinary sleep clinics in the UK/Ireland, which is located at the Mater Private Hospital in Dublin.

According to Dr Crowe, sleep could be considered as an altered state of consciousness, during which there is perceptual disengagement from the environment. Within sleep there are two separate states, which have been defined on the basis of different physiological parameters. These two states, non rapid eye movement (NREM) sleep and rapid eye movement (REM) sleep, exist in nearly all mammals and birds and, surprisingly, are as distinct from one another as each is from wakefulness.

What are NREM and REM Sleep?

NREM (pronounced non REM) sleep is divided into four stages. Stage 1 is very light sleep, usually occurring just after sleep onset; and Stage 4 is very deep sleep, with Stages 2 and 3 in between. REM sleep is so called on account of the bursts of rapid eye movements which occur during this time. The mental activity of REM sleep is associated with dreaming. Another feature of REM sleep is lack of muscle tone which can sometimes persist momentarily into wakefulness if a person suddenly awakens during REM.

A normal healthy adult will enter sleep through Stage 1 and on into Stages 2, 3 and 4. REM sleep does not occur until ninety minutes or so after sleep onset. NREM sleep and REM sleep will then alternate cyclically throughout the night. Deep, or Stage 3 or 4, sleep predominates in the first third of the night and REM sleep in the last third.

The following is a breakdown of the percentages of overall sleep time spent by a young adult in each stage of a normal night's sleep.

- Stage 1 (drowsiness): 2% to 5%
- Stage 2 (light sleep): 45% to 55%
- Stage 3 (deep/slow wave sleep): 3% to 8%
- Stage 4 (deep/slow wave sleep): 10% to 15%
- REM (dream sleep): 20% to 25%

The strongest factor to affect sleep is age. Slow wave sleep is maximal in young children and decreases markedly with age. REM sleep is maintained into old age.

The exact functions of REM and NREM sleep are still not clearly known. Various theories, in relation to different species, have been postulated over the years. These ideas include the restorative role, energy conservation and immobilisation theory. A more recent proposition, though not necessarily universally accepted, is that only core sleep is necessary and that the rest of the sleep is time-filling. Core sleep is thought to be important for brain restitution. It corresponds primarily with deep NREM sleep and some REM sleep.

Circadian Rhythms

When we sleep is influenced by what are known as circadian rhythms. The word circadian is derived from the latin *circa* meaning 'around' and *dies* meaning 'day'. In lay terms, circadian rhythms revolve around a biological clock of roughly twenty-five hours' duration. The underlying principle is that all internal body functions have a direct relationship to each other and are timed to synchronise within about twenty-four to twenty-five hours, regardless of constant darkness or other light conditions.

These rhythms have different patterns depending on the time of day. Examples — apart from sleep and wakefulness —

include body temperature, various hormones and digestive tract activity.

When sleep is examined with reference to circadian body temperature pattern, it is clear that sleep onset is most unlikely to occur when the temperature curve is falling; and waking up occurs more often when body temperature is rising. Peak REM time happens when body temperature is at its lowest. This explains why sleep can be difficult when there is desynchronisation between sleep and body temperature curves, such as occurs in jet lag and shift work. Trying to sleep in a hot environment can be troublesome for the same reason.

Peaks and Valleys

Ever found yourself at mid-afternoon meetings nodding off? The likelihood is that you assumed it was due solely to a bad night's sleep the night before, to boredom, an overly stuffy atmosphere, or the after effects of lunch. In reality, however, the causes may not necessarily be any of those things.

Mid-afternoon dip is extremely common, and is linked to our circadian rhythm cycle. During the 2.30 p.m. to 4.30 p.m. time frame, certain areas of the brain work more sluggishly. In terms of creativity and productivity, therefore, performance during this period tends to be at its lowest. In contrast, late morning tends to be when the creative side of the brain is at its sharpest.

Other areas of the brain, however, tend to function best earlier in the morning. For example, short-term memory tasks (where you've got to remember digits/words) tend to be best then, but deteriorate as the day goes on. However, this is always modulated by the amount of sleep you've had the night before: the less you've had, the more extreme the reaction.

Other Influences of Circadian Rhythms

Circadian rhythms have a bearing on other functions, such as digestion. It is optimum in the morning and at midday, which is why doctors recommend that the biggest meals of the day be taken then.

Circadian rhythms also control body temperature. Body temperature tends to rise gradually during the day, peaks around ten in the evening, plummets during the night and plateaus and then rises again before you wake up. The important thing to remember about the biological clock and body temperature variations is that if you're doing mental performance tasks, the speed at which you can do many of these tasks will increase during the day as body temperature rises. The key influences on the overall level of task performance, therefore, are how much sleep you have had the night before and where you are on the biological clock.

According to Dr Chris Idzikowski, past Chairman of the British Sleep Society and a leading sleep research scientist, there is also some loose evidence that all of us operate on a ninety-minute cycle during the day. Experiments have shown that people will tend to want to eat or nibble food every ninety minutes if left to their own devices, and without the benefit of any light, time or social cues. They show the same cycle pattern with daydreaming.

There are some indications that tasks like study, work or writing are best accomplished in ninety-minute cycles. Other studies have shown that air traffic controllers work best on ninety-minute rotating shifts.

Waking at Night

Finally, apart from REM (dream) sleep occurring on a ninety-minute cycle, you also wake up every hour and a half. When young, you're not aware of this. As you get older, however, those periods of wakefulness get longer. If you're anxious about something, then those are the times you tend to break out of your sleep.

If you do wake up and spend fifteen to twenty minutes awake, the chances are you probably won't get back to sleep until roughly ninety minutes from the time you woke. In such circumstances, it's probably best to give up the battle and instead do something relaxing or creative, like writing or reading.

The same principle applies if you're planning to catch an early morning flight. Simply try to work out when you usually go to sleep and then make your sleeping time a round number of ninety minutes. For example, if you set your alarm to ring within either six hours or seven and a half hours from the time of falling asleep, you'll wake up feeling fresher.

The same principle applies to naps. Duration should always be for variants of ninety minutes, not odd periods such as one and a quarter hours. If you deviate from this formula, the odds are you will still be in a deeper sleep and it will be harder to wake up.

CHAPTER 2

How Much Sleep Do We Need?

When it comes to measuring how much sleep people need, it's really only possible to refer to averages. However, when it comes to determining sleep norms, there does seem to be a correlation between age, body development and actual sleep requirements. The scale is roughly as follows:

◆ babies of two months or less need about sixteen to seventeen hours a day
◆ babies of four months need about ten hours a night, plus two long and one short nap during the day
◆ one-year-olds need thirteen to fourteen hours in twenty-four (usually made up of eleven hours at night and some short and long naps)
◆ children aged between five and fifteen need nine to ten hours
◆ adolescents need about ten hours
◆ adults average about eight hours, but this can vary from as few as four to six hours to as many as nine to ten hours.

Adolescents' sleep needs are not generally recognised, which is causing psycho-social problems, particularly in the United States.

According to Dr Idzikowski, it is difficult to define norms as such. People vary, and they vary throughout their lives. Older people in their seventies may sleep at night for as little as four or five hours (although the average is about six and a half hours). However, whereas they may do rather badly with night-time sleep, they may nap to make up the shortfall during the following day — often without quite realising the extent of that napping.

Assessing Your Needs

The averages given here are only that, however. The real question is: are *you* getting enough sleep? No-one knows how much sleep you really need — it varies from person to person. What matters is how you feel, and the manifestations of poor quality sleep, or sleep deprivation, if any. These include feeling tired, having slower reflexes, poor judgment, lack of energy, bad humour, or having difficulty carrying out lengthy or repetitive tasks. These are just general guidelines, of course. Any one of those could be attributed to other causes!

Identifying a Problem

If you identify positively with the following statements, the likelihood is that you're not doing so well in the sleep stakes, and as a result may be suffering from sleep deprivation:

◆ you often wake up feeling unrefreshed
◆ you don't feel fully alert during the day, are often drowsy, or feel like taking a nap
◆ you tend to have ongoing difficulties with concentration, or learning tasks
◆ you have memory problems
◆ you often find yourself nodding off while driving; while waiting in traffic at a red light; while carrying out monotonous tasks, or while watching television.

The chances are that the above are caused by your having trouble either falling asleep, or staying asleep. Alternatively, you may be getting poor quality sleep, or simply spending insufficient time in bed. Putting up with these situations isn't necessarily serious or injurious to health. But they may in themselves cause anxiety or depression, which can seriously affect quality of life for you and your family.

The acid test is to appraise your own performance. How do you feel? How productive are you? Are you a morning or an evening person? If you think you have a sleeping problem, then the first step is to keep a sleep diary for a few weeks.

Getting Help

If you feel you need help, talk to your GP. He or she may refer you to a sleep clinic for scientific monitoring of your sleep patterns. This is the most accurate way to ascertain the type and quality of your sleep and it can also quantify how much sleep you are getting. It will go some way towards assisting the doctor/therapist to devise the appropriate treatment for you later, should you be unlucky enough to have sleep apnoea, narcolepsy or some other sleep disorder.

During just one night at a sleep clinic, brain wave measurement tests can tell whether someone is asleep, what kinds of sleep he or she is experiencing, and for how long. (See Chapters 3 and 5 for information on sleep disorders and how to get help.)

A Simple Experiment

If you don't have a sleeping problem, but are curious to establish precisely what your sleep requirements are, you can conduct your own private experiment. This is probably best carried out while on holiday, or at least when you are not pressured for time, stressed, or unable to establish a fixed routine. The process is simple, and is designed to pinpoint what time you would wake if left to your own devices, and allowed to respond to your body's needs.

Every night for two weeks, go to bed at the same time, keeping a note of how long you reckon it took to fall asleep and what time you woke. Do not use an alarm clock at any point. This test is designed to establish at what time you would wake *naturally*. Expect to sleep longer than usual for the first few days or so. If you have been working hard, or sleeping less than you should, your body may need a while to make up that deficit.

After two weeks, an overall pattern should emerge. When you look at that pattern, you can work out more accurately what time you should be going to bed and how much sleep you need. You can then adjust your sleeping habits accordingly. If it takes, say, one and a half hours to go asleep, this could indicate a circadian rhythm problem. If that is the case, give up trying to defeat your biological clock and delay your bedtime accordingly.

Actigraphy

Recently, movement detection devices which measure sleep have come into use. The advantage of these is that you don't need to keep a sleep diary. All that's required of the person undergoing sleeping pattern analysis is that he or she wear a device which looks a bit like a wristwatch. Print-outs can then be analysed by a sleep disorders specialist.

Night-Time Awakenings

Before finishing on the subject of how much sleep we need and for how long, a word about night-time awakenings.

Firstly, sporadic night-time awakenings are a normal occurrence. As already pointed out in Chapter 1, All About Sleep, you can expect to wake at least once every ninety minutes during the night. However, unless the wakeful period lasts at least seven minutes, you won't be able to recall it the next morning. This is because memory is affected by sleep. And it is also why we can never be certain of the precise time we fell asleep, and why we tend to be very hazy about events that occurred during the night.

As we get older, night-time awakenings increase in duration. So, from remembering just a couple of awakenings each night as young adults, this increases to many times a night after middle age. This is considered normal. However, patterns are believed to have deviated from the norm if night-time awakenings occur so often that only eighty-five per cent of the time in bed is actually spent asleep. The lower the figure drops after that, the nearer a person gets to being classified an insomniac.

CHAPTER 3

Common Sleep Disorders

Leaving the effects of shift work or jet lag aside, most everyday sleep disturbances are caused by anxiety, or by not being able to cope with the stresses of life. Insomnia is the commonest sleep disorder. Its root cause is usually related specifically to:

◆ anxiety
◆ stress
◆ tension
◆ depression
◆ body clock disorders such as delayed and advanced sleep phase syndrome.

Other common sleep disorders are:

◆ snoring/sleep apnoea
◆ hypersomnia (sleeping too much) due to other causes including narcolepsy
◆ restless legs syndrome
◆ sleep-walking, nightmares and night terrors
◆ bruxism (teeth grinding).

While bruxism is classified as a sleep disorder, it is probably more likely to disturb sleeping partners than the sleepers themselves.

Chapter 5 in this book deals with specialists' comments on and treatments for other common conditions, but here I am going to concentrate on insomnia and its most common causes.

Insomnia

In the real dark night of the soul,
it is always three o'clock in the morning.

F. Scott Fitzgerald

The World Health Organisation defines insomnia as a condition of unsatisfactory quantity and/or quality of sleep, which persists for a considerable period of time. According to Dr Chris Idzikowski, ninety-nine per cent of people suffer from sleeplessness at some time. In itself, this is not a problem. Transient insomnia is not something people should bother trying to treat or cure — there's no need. If there is no underlying physiological or psychological cause, a person's normal sleep pattern will restore itself in due course. Sleeplessness only becomes a problem when it can be described as chronic.

Who Gets Insomnia?

Anything up to half the population suffers from insomnia at some stage in their lives. About five per cent of those will be under thirty; this rises to thirty-five per cent in the over-sixty-five age group. It also affects more women than men.

One theory is that the higher incidence of insomnia in middle-aged and older women is a consequence of long-standing disrupted sleep during child-rearing years: fifteen to twenty-five years later comes the pay back! This theory isn't as unlikely as it may sound. For example, studies of shift workers have shown that these people tend to manifest with sleeping problems *ten years* after stopping shift work.

One theory about sleep problems and older people is that the production of the hormone melatonin — which is produced by the pineal gland in the brain, and regulates our sleep/wake cycles — decreases as we get older. Some scientists believe this is why younger people have fewer problems sleeping than older people. At the time of writing, there is much controversy about the widespread use of commercially manufactured melatonin, particularly in the United States, where it is available as an over-the-counter preparation (see page 27 for more on melatonin).

What is Insomnia?

Insomnia isn't a disease, it's generally a symptom of some other underlying cause. In eighty per cent of insomnia cases seen by GPs, the most common cause is a range of psychological problems such as anxiety and depression. A corollary of this is that if depression isn't at the root of the insomnia, untreated insomnia over a prolonged period can lead to depression.

Doctors divide insomnia into three types:

◆ transient: lasting a few days
◆ short term: up to three weeks
◆ chronic: three weeks or longer.

The causes can in turn be divided into the following seven categories.

1 *Physical* Respiratory problems, including: asthma; hay fever; bronchitis; a cold; sleep apnoea (akin to chronic snoring, and common in middle-aged men who are also overweight); restless legs; tinnitus; some cancers (particularly bone, pancreas and brain cancers); pain caused by toothache, backache, headache; arthritis; a physical injury; food poisoning; menstruation; menopause or pre-menstrual syndrome; hypertension.

2 *Physiological* Day-time napping; strenuous late-night exercise; jet lag; noise; pregnancy; shift work; low blood sugar due to not eating the right food at the right time; sudden weight loss from dieting; digestive disturbances from eating a heavy meal late in the evening.

3 *Psychological* Grief; stress; tension; worry; anticipation; excitement.

4 *Psychiatric* Depression; anxiety; post traumatic stress disorder; any severe psychiatric disorder.

5 *Pharmacological* Alcohol; some anti-depressants; beta-blockers; corticosteroids; theophyline; caffeine and products containing caffeine, such as tea, colas and other fizzy drinks, and chocolate — particularly the rich, dark variety; illicit drugs; nicotine; nasal decongestants; some asthma remedies. Withdrawal from psycho-active drugs can also affect sleep quality.

6 *Environmental* These include over- or under-heating the bedroom; noise in all its manifestations, ranging from traffic to noisy neighbours or a snoring partner; discomfort; allergy to house dust mites; light.

7 *Circadian Rhythm Disorders* These include delayed sleep phase syndrome, where sleep time is very late (common in young people); and advanced sleep phase syndrome, where sleep time is too early (more common in elderly people). These disorders are due to circadian rhythms being out of sync with normal daily life.

Specific Aggravating Factors
Alcohol

Alcohol, a nervous system depressant, can help sleep onset and may initially deepen sleep and decrease REM sleep. But it is usually followed in the second half of the night — as its effects wear off — by increased REM, more disturbed sleep, or perhaps nightmares. The greater the amount of alcohol, the worse the effect.

Like some sleeping pills, alcohol depresses the brain systems that control wakefulness. As its effects wear off, a wake rebound reaction occurs. This causes restlessness and fragmented sleep. It also increases the chances of waking up in the middle of a dream.

Allergic Itch/Skin Disorders

These include eczema, urticaria (hives) and insect bites. These and other allergic skin conditions can conspire to make sure you get a poor night's sleep.

Asthma

Some asthmatics wake during the small hours with distressed breathing. One school of thought is that timing the taking of medication may help. Taking it last thing at night may increase its effectiveness and prevent insomnia. Eliminating environmental/allergic causes of the problem could also help.

Night/Shift Working

Night and shift workers are particularly prone to various digestive disorders. Causes are partly diet related and partly due to upset circadian rhythms, which in turn interfere with the digestive system. This is further aggravated by factors such as greasy food and eating rich meals too close to bedtime.

Endocrine Diseases

These problems include diabetes (with thirst) and hypoglycaemia.

Frequency (the desire to urinate)

Causes may include early diabetes; sleep apnoea; over-consumption of alcohol, tea or coffee; prostate trouble in men; cystitis or the onset of menopause — in women — which can cause bladder problems; and, as mentioned below, treatment with diuretics.

Heart Disease

This may be combined with chest pain or respiratory problems, leading to breathlessness. It also has links to sleep apnoea.

High Blood Pressure

This is a related problem. Patients being treated for this condition with certain beta-blockers may have particular difficulties, as these drugs can create a stimulating rather than sedating effect. Beta-blockers can also cause nightmares. Diuretics, another type treatment for heart disease and hypertension, can lead to urinary frequency at night (see above), especially if taken late in the day.

Older People and Sleeping Problems

The most common causes of insomnia in older people include the types of medical conditions listed earlier in this chapter, combined with the side-effects of the medications used to treat those conditions. In addition, the incidence of sleep apnoea and restless legs syndrome increases with age. Menopause can also affect the quality of sleep in older women.

Sleep changes as we get older. This is a normal physiological phenomenon. Some of those changes are caused by the variations in our circadian rhythms becoming less marked.

Older people have much less deep sleep. The awakening threshold also decreases with age. For example, a noise level sufficient to wake up a seventy-year-old will only cause a transient shift to light sleep in a twenty-five-year-old. Medical conditions and the taking of various medications are more common with increased age. As a result, the sleep of healthy and previously good sleepers can become fragile, and frequent awakenings more common — anything up to 150 times a night. (Young adults, by comparison, may only waken briefly about five times a night.)

Assuming there are no underlying medical conditions as described above, or the more common conditions of old age such as arthritis or rheumatism, then frequent awakenings shouldn't be considered abnormal. Staying awake for long periods is abnormal, however.

Sometimes the problem may be self-induced. For example, it's very common for older people to make up for a bad night's sleep by retiring at 10 p.m. or earlier, and then remaining in bed until 9 o'clock the next morning. Aspiring to achieve eleven hours' sleep in such circumstances is unrealistic: the longer you stay in bed, the *less* likely you are to fill that time with sleep.

Dr Crowe's advice to older people who complain of fragmented sleep is to spend eight hours in bed at most, if their actual sleep requirement is, say, six hours. If they feel tired in between, the advice is to take a nap rather than trying to get as much sleep as possible in one go at night.

Restless Legs Syndrome

This is a common cause of sleeping problems in older people. It is usually associated with a condition called periodic limb movements during sleep. Restless legs syndrome is described as an uncomfortable sensation in the legs, associated with an irresistible urge to move around. It is usually worst in the evening, and can stop the sufferer from getting to sleep.

Periodic leg movements consist of brief, repetitive leg jerks occurring during sleep. These are often, but not necessarily, linked to awakenings — although the patient may not know why he or she has woken up.

According to Dr Crowe, restless legs syndrome can be associated with certain medical conditions like anaemia, diabetes or chronic renal failure; so it is clearly important to deal with any underlying causes first. It can be a very distressing condition, having a major negative impact on a person's general quality of life.

Some people will respond well to taking more exercise, or hot baths; others say it makes the condition worse. Often the condition will come and go for no particular reason. Certain medications can help. Others, such as anti-depressants, can make it worse, so discuss the problem with your GP.

Jet Lag

The jet lag that comes about from long-haul flying is inextricably linked with upset to our circadian rhythms. It generally only becomes an issue where flights last five hours or more. Although there is some debate about this, it's usually worse going from west to east. It's *not* a factor, however, with flights from the northern to the southern hemisphere, as long as both the departure and destination points are in the same time zone; a trip from London to Johannesburg shouldn't create a jet lag problem, for example.

The main cause of jet lag is the biological disruption which occurs from flying across time zones faster than the body can adjust. Symptoms may include chronic fatigue for days after arrival; irregularities in bowel movements; indigestion and loss of appetite; daytime sleepiness; headaches; irritability; disorientation, or fuzziness; difficulty concentrating or motivating yourself for energetic tasks; becoming irrational or unreasonable; and most importantly of all in the context of this book, difficulties in getting to sleep, coupled with frequent awakenings/broken sleep. All of these combine to cause night-time alertness and day-time drowsiness. Quite a cocktail!

Symptoms are aggravated because of the mismatching between your body clock and the local time at the destination. The circadian system is unable to adjust immediately, and a certain inertia manifests instead.

For example, following a six-hour flight from west to east, you may feel tired, and your ability to carry out a number of reasoning tasks will be at its lowest from 6 a.m. to 2 p.m. on the new time scale. On the other hand, following a flight east to west, by 6 p.m. local time, your circadian rhythms will dictate that your body is ready for bed, while your mind and the environment around you dictate that you should be active and alert. The consequent loss of sleep from this kind of biological disruption may affect your ability to function well, while the *quality* of that sleep will also change. And so it goes on.

Some experts reckon you need to allow one day's recovery time for every time zone crossed, in order to regain normal rhythm and energy levels. In theory, crossing eight time zones — say, from California to London — could take eight days to re-synchronise. Generally, however, jet lag symptoms decline after about three days, as the body clock and biorhythms synchronise with the new time zone.

Reducing the Effects of Jet Lag

Generally, children under three suffer least and adults with very fixed routines suffer most. Night owls find it easier to go west and larks (early risers) find it easier to go east. The effects of jet lag can be greatly reduced, provided you follow a few fairly simple routines.

Exercise should be part of your daily routine anyway, but it's even more important if you're about to take a long-haul flight. Being moderately fit can help lessen the impact of jet lag.

Alcohol consumed while you're flying is two to three times stronger than the equivalent amount consumed on the ground. If you're already hungover, or sleep deprived, before you begin the flight, then by drinking on the aircraft you will multiply the hangover effect awaiting you on arrival at your destination. The risk of hangover is greatly increased with even fairly moderate alcohol consumption while flying. Alcohol also exacerbates the dehydration problem associated with air travel.

Unless you're lucky enough to be flying business class, aircraft eating and sleeping conditions will probably be very cramped. Sitting in such conditions puts additional pressure on your stomach, so digestive functions are constrained. Eat as little as possible on flights for that reason. At least avoid rich, fatty foods, which are more difficult to digest than other foods.

Be judicious about your consumption of coffee, tea and chocolate (all of which contain caffeine). These strong stimulants will almost certainly interfere with your sleep. And even if in-flight caffeine *before* sleeping doesn't delay the onset of sleep, it may trigger awakenings later.

As airlines increasingly trim running costs, in-flight air quality decreases pro rata, unless you happen to be seated in business class. The flight crew won't always acquiesce, but you've nothing to lose by requesting that the pilot increase aircraft oxygen intake. If you're stuck on a long and crowded flight and the air quality is foul, it will help you feel better.

Existing colds and flu's are made worse by long-haul flights. Dry aircraft atmosphere and stale air can also cause headaches, dry skin, dry nose and throat. The importance of drinking lots of water cannot be emphasised strongly enough. Whatever your normal daily quota is, double it! In order not to disturb the crew or other passengers, carry your own supply of bottled water in your hand luggage.

Preparing your body in advance for the daily routine of your destination will greatly help reduce jet lag. Therefore, once on board, set your watch for your destination time and plan your eating and sleeping routine for the next twenty-four hours, according to the destination timetable.

It's probably unnecessary to say it, but it's not a good idea to take a long-haul flight without a good night's sleep before departure. Sleeping on most aircraft is not that easy, so going into deficit early on in the process is best avoided.

If you have to take a night flight west to east, change into loose, warm, comfortable clothes and prepare for sleep as soon after take-off as possible. Remove shoes and anything tight fitting; leave instructions not to be woken, and forget about in-flight meals. Eye shades, neck pillows and ear plugs may all help your battle to get to sleep. If you don't have your own, the flight crew may supply them, so do ask.

If it's a daytime flight, take as much exercise as possible. Usually a combination of stretching exercises in your seat and walking up and down the aircraft will help.

If you're on a very long flight with a stop-over, get off the plane and stretch your legs. Better still, take a shower if you can. It will freshen you up and help get your blood circulation — already constricted by long periods sitting still — going again.

On Arrival

Take some gentle exercise at the start of the new day at your destination. After that, some experts recommend going to bed and sleeping for one and a half to three hours (or multiples of ninety minutes). Use an alarm clock or a wake-up call to make sure you don't sleep much longer than that. Don't take other naps during the days immediately after the journey, as they will confuse the body about what is night time, consequently slowing down the adaptation process.

Some experts believe that exposing the eyes to bright sunlight at critical times of the day soon after arrival can help, as bright sunlight exposure for one hour in the morning may accelerate the re-synchronisation process. If you have completed a west to east flight, say London to Hong Kong, you should expose yourself to sunlight in the mid- to late-afternoon on the first day. On the second day, expose yourself to light at midday. And on days three and four, go out in the sunshine during late morning (10 to 11 a.m.).

If you have flown from London to Los Angeles, you should get as much light as possible in the late afternoon/early evening on day one, and late evening on days two to four.

The general rule is that light late in the day makes the circadian rhythms late (i.e. later to sleep is later to wake). Light early in the day pushes the rhythm earlier (i.e. earlier to sleep is earlier to wake). The more time zones you cross, the longer it takes to move the rhythms into synchrony with the new bedtime.

Melatonin

The jury is still out on the usefulness of taking melatonin supplements as a way of helping jet lag sufferers reset their circadian rhythms. Some people swear by it; others say it makes them depressed.

Melatonin is a natural hormone, produced by the pineal gland in the brain at night. It is activated by darkness, increases during the night, and then decreases as morning approaches and light intensifies. It is believed to have certain links with immune system performance, but one of its main functions is to set the internal biological clock that governs our cycles or rhythms. Clearly, long-haul flights can disrupt that dark/light exposure and sleep patterns can go haywire. A small dose of commercially produced melatonin taken just before bedtime may be a useful way to reset the sleep/wake cycle.

A relatively new product, the side effects of commercially produced melatonin are not fully known. At the time of writing, it is not available in certain countries, although it is widely available in the US, where it may be bought as an over-the-counter preparation.

Other Medications

There are a number of other 'no jet lag' preparations on the market, including homeopathic remedies, which are taken in extremely low dosages. These products do not contain melatonin, and are popular with some experienced long-haul flight passengers.

A recent study showed that seventy per cent of sleep disorders specialists do not take sleeping pills even for jet lag. Avoid sleeping pills if you possibly can. However, small doses of a short-acting hypnotic may help on the second night following arrival. Generally speaking, sleep deprivation guarantees sleep on the first night.

Night/Shift Working

Changing work practices in service industries worldwide now mean that more and more people are working the kind of hours that do not coincide with their normal circadian rhythms. Because they are out of sync, shift workers in general — and night workers in particular — may suffer sleeping problems such as insomnia as a result. They also tend to have a higher rate of illness generally, especially heart disease and digestive disorders, and they are more prone to accidents.

Circadian rhythms are one of life's immutable forces. You can't fool them, and it's difficult to change them. As previously mentioned, they regulate our physiological and behavioural functions on roughly a twenty-five hour basis.

As you will know by now, our sleep and wake patterns, body temperature, hormones, performance, moods, digestion and other bodily functions are all genetically programmed to take place at certain times. As a result, certain universal rules apply. For example, body temperature is at its highest at around 5 p.m. and then it starts to drop.

Alertness and performance follow the same pattern. For someone working through the night, where psycho-motor functions are crucial, the importance of being fully awake is obvious. Drivers, pilots, machinery operators, medical staff, police and power station workers all need to be extra vigilant around this time.

The problems shift workers experience are something akin to jet lag. The combination of adjusting to changing work shifts, sleeping in a brighter room than normal, external noise and daily life going on around them — result in disrupted sleep, and less of it.

According to Dr Catherine Crowe, nobody ever completely adjusts to frequent shift changes. Day sleep after night work tends to be two hours shorter than night sleep. The shortening is primarily taken from Stage 2 as well as REM (dreaming) sleep. Deep, or Stages 3 and 4, sleep does not appear to be affected. On the good news front, Dr Crowe adds that many workers will make up at least some of their lost sleep time on their days off.

Do's and Don'ts for Shift Workers

If you're a permanent night worker (doing five continuous nights at a stretch), you are probably better off than someone doing alternating shifts, because then you can stay with the same eating and sleeping rhythms even on your days off. Although this may be ideal in physiological terms, in social and family terms that kind of discipline is difficult, if not impossible, to adhere to. Either way, the important thing is to stay with the same eating rhythms and try to sleep the usual length of time.

Following a particular bedtime routine is especially important for shift workers, whose attempts to fall asleep and stay asleep face much greater challenges than conventional sleepers. It helps to follow a few basic rules, such as:

- go to bed as soon as possible after returning from work
- avoid any stimulants such as tea, coffee, chocolate or colas for four hours between finishing work and heading for bed (stimulants make it harder to get to sleep, and staying asleep even harder)
- do not smoke for the same reason. Nicotine is a strong stimulant. And apart from all the other health reasons for not smoking, studies have shown that smokers sleep 30 minutes a night *less* than non-smokers. So given that shift workers sleep between five and seven hours less a week anyway, if you are a shift worker and a smoker, you are making yourself doubly vulnerable to sleep deprivation.

Try and get your brain used to the idea of shutting down against strong 'wake up' daylight signals, by doing things like wearing sunglasses on the way home and using dimmer switch lighting in the room you're relaxing in before going to bed. Be careful what you eat before going to sleep. Take something fairly light and digestible. Other general dietary recommendations for shift workers include following a diet high in carbohydrates and protein, and low in fried, fatty foods, or any other foods that are hard to digest.

Block out street, traffic or other environmental noise by running a fan or keep the radio on turned down low. If you don't already have one, consider installing an answering machine to prevent the telephone waking you up. Either install a dark blind in the bedroom to block out daylight, or alternatively wear the kind of eye shades airlines dispense to long-haul flight passengers.

If you're on changing shifts, a short-acting sleeping pill can help reset your circadian rhythms if you're having trouble getting to sleep, or staying asleep. It may be useful for helping to break the sleep disordered cycle, but don't get dependent either on the *idea* of sleeping pills or the pills themselves. Remember, they will lose their effect in a few weeks anyway. Be careful not to mix sleeping pills with either alcohol or anti-histamines.

Valerian is a good alternative to sleeping pills for dealing with mild insomnia. It is widely available in pharmacies and health food stores. You don't need a prescription, and it's a lot cheaper than sleeping pills. See pages 87–97 for information on this and other herbal remedies.

High or moderate physical fitness seems to reduce sleepiness during night shifts and improve sleep quality. The best time to exercise is some time during the afternoon, i.e. immediately after the sleep period.

If your circadian rhythms have gone seriously haywire as a result of periods of shift working, bright light therapy as described later in the book may help. Light boxes are fairly widely available and can be either bought or hired.

The foregoing is by no means a definitive list. Some of the steps for getting a good night's sleep, set out on pages 39–44, may be applied equally well by night/shift workers.

Snoring

Up to one in five adults snore badly enough to drive those sharing a bedroom with them to distraction. Sometimes it causes insomnia in the unfortunate sleeping partner. Men snore more than women, and snoring is aggravated by lying on one's back or by being overweight. Age, alcohol and the use of sleeping pills or other sedatives are also contributory factors.

The good news for snorers, however, is that simple snoring is not believed to cause any health problems. Sleep apnoea is, of course, another matter; reports of a particular kind of snoring may point to this potentially serious condition. If snoring is interspersed with snorting or pauses, think of sleep apnoea. Likewise, if it is associated with unexplained daytime sleepiness, it should be further investigated. Daytime sleepiness can be quite subtle. If you have a tendency to fall asleep regularly in quiet situations, such as watching television, you may have sleep apnoea. But check that you are not sleep deprived for other reasons.

Dr Iain Gleadhill, a consultant physician specialising in respiratory disorders and sleep apnoea, says surgery can sometimes be effective in reducing snoring if there is an abnormality of the nose or palate, but it is certainly not a guaranteed cure. The pros and cons of surgery have to be considered on an individual basis.

Dr Gleadhill advises the following steps for patients whose snoring is causing upset or embarrassment:

- try to learn to sleep on your side (put a tennis ball in a sock and pin that sock to whatever you are wearing in bed; roll over and you wake up, or else go back onto your side)
- if nasal congestion or catarrh is causing the problem, have it treated
- if you're overweight, set about a weight reduction programme
- avoid alcohol near bedtime
- stop smoking.

There are a number of other possible measures you can try. A plastic device, which keeps the nasal passages open during sleep, cures snoring for some people. Alternatively, you can buy another device which is applied externally (on the bridge of the nose). Both are available from pharmacies. An oral appliance which looks a bit like a mouth guard, or gum shield, is a new development which may help snorers. Worn at night, it holds the lower jaw and tongue forward. If you're taking sleeping tablets, cut them out — they only make snoring worse.

If all else fails, buy ear plugs for your partner. You could also consider whether one of you should sleep in another room, for one or two nights a week, to avoid a build-up of fatigue in the unfortunate non-snorer.

Sleep Apnoea Syndrome

The word apnoea derives from the Greek, 'want of breath'. While the condition is not new, general awareness of it is fairly new. Unlike other sleep disorders, such as insomnia, it doesn't come and go — if you have it, it will stay with you until it's treated.

Sleep apnoea goes hand in hand with chronic snoring, gasping and choking for air. People with sleep apnoea don't breathe properly while they're asleep, and therefore don't get enough oxygen. They're a bit like someone at the bottom of a swimming pool who has to rise to the surface every time they need to breathe. During sleep, they come to the surface of consciousness anything up to 600 times a night with gasping attacks. Because breathing is irregular or difficult (they can stop breathing for up to 110 seconds), levels of oxygen in the blood can drop drastically. This may result in rapid changes in heart rate and blood pressure.

The effect of these episodes is to give sufferers very poor quality sleep. Deep (restorative) sleep becomes a virtual impossibility. The next day, they feel as if they have hardly slept at all, so, naturally, the quality of their mood and overall performance during waking hours suffers dramatically. Falling asleep during the day is common. As a result, the perception of these patients by their peers in business, work, social, or academic life can be quite negative.

People with sleep apnoea are up to five times more likely either to be involved in, or actually cause, a car accident. It's inextricably linked to both the respiratory and cardiovascular systems. Sleep-disordered breathing may cause hypertension, and the condition can increase the likelihood of heart attacks and strokes.

Who Suffers from It?

Dr Crowe recalls case histories such as one businessman who not only fell asleep during telephone conversations with clients, but also started to *snore* while still on the phone! Another man remembered falling asleep standing up, while pushing his child on a park swing. And a third, a truck driver, reported incidents of falling asleep at the wheel while driving.

Sleep apnoea is relatively uncommon in women. The typical profile is a middle-aged man, overweight, with a receding chin and short neck, but these are, of course, only general pointers. He may also be a smoker, which may aggravate the condition. And if he combines all of these factors with drinking alcohol (which can interfere with breathing patterns), he may be setting himself up for real trouble.

Sleep apnoea can wreck marriages and relationships. Snoring is bad enough, but people with sleep apnoea also undergo personality changes as a result of being chronically tired and lacking in energy. They may suffer memory loss and irritability. To add to their misery, they may have sexual difficulties (such as impotence), ulcers, morning headaches and depression. They may also suffer from frequency (the desire to urinate during the night).

Very often, an undiagnosed person with sleep apnoea will mistakenly eat high calorie foods, such as chocolate, to give themselves an energy boost. Not only does this not work, but they may also put on weight as a result. As being overweight is linked to the cause of the condition in the first place, unfortunately they end up making an already chronic problem even worse.

Although rare, sleep apnoea can also occur in babies. Some experts believe there is a link between Sudden Infant Death Syndrome (cot death) and sleep apnoea, but this would only be in a minority of cases.

Children can also suffer from the condition. Some of them snore, even though that isn't normal for children — unless they have a cold. Others make squeaky noises or have difficulty breathing. Contributory factors include enlarged tonsils, adenoid trouble and being overweight. Night sweating, particularly of the head and neck, may also be a sign. Like adults, these children may suffer from daytime sleepiness, sluggishness, poor concentration, memory loss and impaired intellectual performance. But over-activity, especially in pre-teenage years, is probably more common.

Diagnosis

Suspicion of the condition may be arrived at as a result of a combination of the patient's description of symptoms and complaints/verification from a partner. This can be confirmed by seeking the advice of a sleep disorders specialist, and having tests carried out in a sleep clinic.

Treatment

The positive news about sleep apnoea is that it is eminently treatable.

With moderate to severe sleep obstructive sleep apnoea, the most effective treatment is delivered by a device known as CPAP (continuous positive airway pressure, pronounced *see-pap*.) This regulatory respiratory device effectively keeps the upper airway open during sleep, while pressure from an air compressor forces air through the nasal passages and into the airway. The device includes a mask to cover the nose and is put on last thing at night. Whereas the whole thing looks cumbersome and restrictive, it is, apparently, surprisingly comfortable and over two-thirds of patients who start will use it long term.

The benefits of this treatment are apparent within days. Previously sleepy patients feel as if a cloud has been lifted from their heads — often in a dramatic fashion. Many say CPAP has changed their lives.

Both conventional and laser surgery may correct the physical causes of sleep apnoea, including enlarged tonsils or adenoids; nasal polyps or other growths; a long soft palate; or a deviated septum, from old nose injuries. It works for about half of all sleep apnoea cases. It is more likely to work in the less severe cases, where obstruction is due to a single cause and obesity is not a factor, so patients should be carefully selected. All patients with sleep apnoea syndrome who have surgery should have a follow-up sleep recording four to six months later, to ensure that the condition is under control.

Losing weight and getting fit are highly recommended for all sleep apnoea patients, in addition to other specific treatments.

Practical Steps for Sufferers

If sleep apnoea is suspected, a patient should be evaluated in a sleep clinic and a treatment plan drawn up. If mild sleep apnoea is the cause, the following practical steps can be taken. (These recommendations have been designed by the American Sleep Disorders Association, for sleep apnoea sufferers.)

Obesity/overweight can be contributory factors. Even partial weight loss may improve breathing, and therefore sleep quality. Avoid alcohol within two hours of bedtime. Alcohol depresses breathing and makes apnoeas more frequent and severe. It also seems to trigger apnoeas in people who would otherwise merely snore. Medications prescribed for headaches, anxiety and depression can affect sleep and breathing. Check with your doctor before taking them.

Sleep on your side. Some people suffer from sleep apnoea only when on their backs. To make sure you stay on your side, place a pillow behind your back, or use the tennis ball technique described on page 32.

Medications to relieve congestion of the nose may be helpful in reducing snoring and the likelihood of apnoea.

Narcolepsy

The symptoms of this neurological sleep disorder range from excessive daytime sleepiness, to cataplexy, hypnagogic hallucinations and sleep paralysis. These symptoms can appear all at once, or develop over many years.

It affects about one in 5,000 of the population, men and women equally. Although it can appear at any age, it tends to present for the first time during the teens and twenties. It is a condition for life, is genetic in origin and has a tendency to run in some families.

The symptoms are due to excessive sleep and poorly regulated dream (REM) sleep.

Day-Time Sleepiness

Features of this are a mixture of inappropriate sleep attacks — literally falling asleep on the spot — often with no warning; a strong desire for more sleep; and a state of sub-alertness or feeling constantly under par. This mix varies, and depends on the individual, but overall it leads to a sensation of significant sleepiness during the day.

REM-Related Phenomena

1 *Cataplexy* Features of this are sudden loss of muscle power, usually brought on by emotions such as laughing or anger. It can affect either all the muscles or just the jaw, for example. While in the cataplectic state, people are not actually asleep, but may go on to sleep. Cataplexy occurs in most, but not all, narcoleptics.

2 *Hypnogogic Hallucinations* These occur just before falling asleep at night, or during naps. The episodes can include feeling as if someone is present in the room, perceiving small animals, or feeling pressure on the bed.

3 *Sleep Paralysis* This features waking during REM sleep, where paralysis normally occurs; the patient is not completely switched on to wakefulness, and so cannot move or talk for a brief time. It is a distressing condition when not understood.

Narcoleptic patients also sometimes suffer from disturbed night sleep. The recommendations elsewhere in the book for insomnia should help.

Treatments

For day-time sleepiness, stimulant drugs including Dexedrine and Ritalin are usually used, but others are available and being developed. REM sleep-related phenomena are treated with anti-depressants in small doses, as they suppress REM sleep. Treatment of REM symptoms is usually quite satisfactory.

Treatment of sleepiness leads to much improved quality of life, but is unlikely to bring the patient completely back to normal. One or two naps of less than an hour are usually still necessary.

Narcolepsy sufferers are also more likely to suffer from sleep apnoea syndrome and periodic leg movements in sleep than the normal population. If sleepiness increases for no obvious reason, either of these may be the cause and should be treated in their own right.

Bruxism (Teeth Grinding)

Night-time teeth grinding is reasonably common — figures indicate anywhere between one in twenty and one in five of the population. Its causes are unknown. It comes and goes, with each episode lasting for about ten seconds.

Sufferers aren't usually aware that they are grinding their teeth, and are probably made aware of it by their sleeping partners. Following extended periods of teeth grinding, they may experience facial pain, but that tends to happen only in severe cases.

A visit to the dentist may turn up evidence of damage to the teeth, but bruxism doesn't affect quality of sleep as such. However, in order to avoid damage to teeth, it is best avoided. The wearing of a plastic mouth guard over the teeth at night is the usual treatment.

Day-time teeth grinding is another matter. Unlike its nocturnal cousin, it is related to stress, and can be treated by biofeedback or other relaxation methods.

CHAPTER 4

How to Get a Better Night's Sleep

Early to bed and early to rise makes a man healthy, wealthy and unfortunately a bit of a social outcast.

Anon

I f you have sleeping difficulties from time to time, and have already established that the causes are not serious enough to require medical intervention, a few simple steps should be sufficient to rectify your problems.

Some of the do's and don'ts that apply to helping you get a good night's sleep read like an anti-fun regime — and in some ways they are. But insomnia — even for a short period — is no fun either. Only you can decide if getting a good-quality night's sleep merits the sacrifices you may have to make to change your lifestyle.

Twenty-Three Steps to a Good Night's Sleep

Points one and two will well and truly put a dint in your social life, and, if followed to the letter, would close down half the restaurants and pubs in the world. But here goes anyway …

1   Despite the night-cap myth, consumption of alcohol is not recommended. Whereas it may help *induce* sleep, it may also make it more fragile, with frequent awakening or lack of deep sleep the result. You should avoid alcohol within

two hours of bedtime, and before that period, keep consumption moderate. Alcohol is metabolised at the rate of about one drink per hour. So, if you consume four drinks, you'll need four hours to metabolise them. This is no problem if you start drinking early in the evening, but a completely different story if much later than that.

2   You shouldn't consume tea, coffee, chocolate (which contains caffeine), cocoa, colas, or fizzy drinks containing cola within four to six hours before bedtime. On those occasions where you deviate from these rules, don't be surprised if you suffer broken sleep. Both alcohol and caffeine interfere with deep sleep. (They don't have a universally negative effect on sleep, however — these are general guidelines and averages.)

3   Appetite suppressants and many commonly used drugs and over-the-counter preparations for headaches, hay fever and colds may contain caffeine or other stimulating ingredients. Check the ingredients before taking medication in the hours before bedtime.

4   To put the importance of keeping regular bedtime hours into perspective, research has shown that the population at large takes at least a week to adjust to the effects of the summer/winter clock time change. So the good sleep message is to keep regular bedtime hours, if at all possible rising at the same time every day. Avoid sleeping in at weekends, except occasionally, unless you want to run the risk of 'Sunday night insomnia'.

If your routine goes out of sync at holiday times, or if you do suffer from Sunday night insomnia, the simplest way to readjust your body clock is to set an alarm clock early in the morning and force yourself to get up at that time — *regardless* of how much sleep you've had the night before. Shortening your sleep will increase the pressure for sleep the following night. By getting up at the same time the following morning, you will be reinforcing the synchronisation of the body clock with the sleep/wake cycle. You should soon find that you are going to sleep at the right time and waking up when you want.

5   Adjust your total sleep time to fit your needs. Because we all have different requirements, that could be as little as four hours, or as many as nine. (Former British prime minister Margaret Thatcher reputedly needed only four to five hours. Einstein needed ten.) Check pages 12–14 for ways of identifying whether or not you are meeting your psychological and physiological sleep requirements.

6   Take regular daily exercise, preferably in the late afternoon or early evening. Early morning exercise doesn't have any bearing on that night's sleep quality as such, although it will impact on your general fitness. As a rule, fitness is a factor in overall sleep quality. See pages 48–9 for details about how much, when and what types of exercise to take.

7   Set aside time in the period after dinner — but *not* immediately before your bedtime ritual — to plan the next day. Make a list of tasks, or organise yourself so that you don't stay awake in bed planning the next day's activities.

8   Keep the bedroom cool. Ideally, the temperature should be between 62 and 65 degrees Fahrenheit, and no higher than 75 degrees. If you're not bothered by pollution, noise or draughts, then by all means keep the bedroom window open in winter. There are no other hard and fast rules about ventilation. The bed, on the other hand, should be warm if you're the type of person who is sensitive to cold.

9   Don't eat heavy meals within two hours before bedtime, but don't go to bed hungry either. See pages 47–8 for specific recommendations on diet/eating.

10 Allow yourself one hour before bedtime to unwind. It is best not to watch television or do anything else that over-stimulates the brain. For example, try not to have a major discussion about important issues — or worse, a row — with

your partner or another family member immediately before going to bed.

11 Use that hour to follow a relaxing bedtime ritual — perhaps having a warm bath or reading.

12 Only be prepared to go to sleep when you are drowsy. Otherwise you are just creating the opportunity to lie awake worrying about it.

13 Make judicious use of herbal remedies — use an aromatherapy burner to burn lavender oil in the bedroom an hour before bedtime. Or place a few drops of lavender oil on your pillow. You might like to consider buying a hops pillow, provided you don't have a history of depression. (Hops may be contra-indicated for depression.)

14 Don't just lie there: if you don't fall asleep after about thirty minutes, do something else. Try playing a relaxation tape (widely available in pharmacies). If that doesn't work, it's better to leave the bedroom and engage in a quiet activity like reading, or listening to BBC Radio 4 (some people swear by it!) until you feel drowsy.

   If, on the other hand, you have a tendency to wake in the early hours of the morning for no apparent reason (common in women around the time of menopause, and in older people), try not to panic about it. Regard it as a bonus; make use of the time by doing something creative — writing letters, practising a hobby, painting, knitting, catching up on the ironing, whatever you find either productive or relaxing.

15 Psychologically, it's best to associate your bedroom with sex and/or sleeping only. During the day, do your telephoning, work, worrying, eating, playing with your computer, or watching television, somewhere else.

16 Likewise, don't spend too much time in bed when you're not sleeping.

17 If you can't, or don't want, to take a warm bath as part of your pre-bedtime ritual, try the old Chinese remedy of

soaking your feet in warm water for twenty minutes before going to bed. Then massage each foot with oil before finally going to sleep.

18 If sex isn't possible for one reason or another (and even if it is!), get your partner to give you a massage too.

19 Avoid daytime naps if you can.

20 If you're one of those people who suddenly puts on or loses weight, don't be surprised if your usual sleep pattern is affected. Fragmented sleep may result from weight loss, whereas long and continuous sleep may result from weight gain. Difficulties in falling asleep, or staying asleep, are the most commonly reported symptoms reported by those who have enrolled in weight reduction programmes. People suffering from anorexia nervosa report something similar. It is not clear whether changes in nutrition status/deficiencies, or altered mood swings, are the root cause.

21 If you use sleeping pills, do not take them every night. You will invariably sleep worse the following night. Expect this, and *don't* take another one. If you have to take them more frequently, a good tip is to keep only one beside the bed for emergencies. Keep the rest locked in a drawer, or somewhere inconvenient to get at. Because the process of having to get out of bed to find them will wake you up, you are much less likely to miscalculate the dosage. Going through this obstacle course means you are also a bit less likely to become dependent on sleeping pills. If you are taking a sleeping pill, it's best to take it before bed, because if taken during the night, it may cause a hangover effect the next day.

22 Contrary to what you might expect, it is not a good idea to overcompensate for one night's sleeplessness by going to bed extra early, or sleeping longer, the next. One night of normal sleep is usually sufficient to make up the deficit. The second night's sleep will be of better quality anyway.

23 Finally, try and be philosophical. Accept an occasional bad night's sleep as part of life. It's a normal, healthy adjustment to changing circumstances, or environmental conditions. After all, you can always use this non-sleeping time for doing something relaxing or creative. Unless your insomnia is both frequent and severely disabling, regard these episodes as a gift of time.

Essential Oils

To achieve a good night's sleep, add six to eight drops of a mix of essential oils to a warm bath. That mix might include lavender, Roman chamomile, sweet marjoram and sandalwood.

Essential oils are extremely strong and are quickly absorbed by the skin. Evidence of this is the speed with which traces appear on exhaled breath. Treat them with respect — they can be very powerful. If you are pregnant, or think you might be, proceed with caution, and seek the advice of a properly qualified aromatherapist.

You also need to be careful about using essential oils on older people who are sick, and on children; half the normal dose may be appropriate for ill, older people, and for children under seven to eight stone (around fifty kilos). Use a quarter of the normal dose for children under four stone (around thirty kilos).

Essential oils are widely available in health food stores and pharmacies. For therapeutic use, buy only brands featuring the scientific name. From a sleep therapy point of view, the most useful ones are:

◆ lavender (*Lavandula angustifolia*), probably the most popular, though not the cheapest essential oil when of therapeutic quality. It has wonderful healing properties
◆ sweet marjoram (*Origanum majorana*), which creates a warm, relaxed feeling. This is a different plant from Spanish

marjoram, which is a species of thyme (*Thymus mastichina*)
and has quite different properties

◆ Roman chamomile (*Chamaemelum nobile*), which gives a
great feeling of warmth and relaxation

◆ geranium (*Pelargonium graveolens*), which helps counteract
nervous tension

◆ sandalwood (*Santalum album*), which is popular with men
and has a lovely, velvety fragrance

◆ neroli (*Citrus aurantium*, var. *amara*), which specifically
helps problems including insomnia; it is a very expensive
oil

◆ mandarin (*Citrus reticulata*), which is also very calming.

To increase the effect, blend two or more of the above oils
together.

Your Bedroom

The wrong kind of bedroom can have a detrimental effect on
sleep quality. There are a number of aspects you should
consider to try and create the ideal bedroom environment.

Because certain types of allergies can interfere with your
sleep, it's a good idea to minimise contributory factors in the
bedroom. If you are asthmatic and think you may be allergic to
the house dust mite, reduce their breeding ground possibilities
by removing heavily upholstered chairs and carpets; replace
these with metal/wooden furniture and wooden or tiled floors.
Buy house dust mite-proof mattress, duvet and pillow covers,
and remove dust by cleaning bedroom surfaces regularly with a
cloth and soapy water. If you are allergic to animal dander, keep
pets out of the bedroom at all times.

High temperatures can lead to disturbances in the quality
of sleep, whereas low temperatures apparently do not.
Whenever practical, keep bedrooms ventilated while sleeping.
Hot, stuffy air may block your nose and sinuses and lead to a

dry throat, headache or tickly cough. Any one of these can disrupt your night's sleep. If opening a window is not an option, and if you suffer from either asthma or bronchitis, try placing a humidifier, or a wet towel, on central heating radiators before going to bed.

Keep the bedroom dark. If you are sensitive to it, light may wake you up before you have had a full night's sleep. Similarly, if you are the type of person who wakes during the night to go to the toilet, keep a torch beside the bed and use that instead of a bright bedroom/bathroom light to find your way. The effect of the latter may be to wake you up so much that it then takes a long time to get back to sleep.

Keep the room as quiet as possible. This may necessitate removing alarm clocks, turning off noisy radiators, or even installing double glazing to eliminate traffic noise. Consider installing an ioniser in the bedroom. These are fairly widely available and not too expensive. If you also happen to suffer from asthma or arthritis, then you'll reap a double benefit.

Bad beds can cause backache, in itself a common cause of sleep loss. Bad back or not, a firm, level and supported mattress is the ideal option. If you can afford it, buy the best quality bed, with an orthopaedic mattress. Otherwise, place a large sheet of plywood under the mattress. Ideally, this should be about 1 in (2.5 cm) thick and should be the same dimensions as the base, i.e. flush with the mattress.

When it comes to pillows, the advice seems to be that less is more, so sleep on the flattest pillow you can bear. Most important, however, is comfort, so use your common sense to decide what suits you best.

Smells of food or cigarette smoke can also interfere with quality of sleep. Make sure to remove any food remnants from the bedroom before you retire for the night. Not only does smoking create a lousy smell that clings to clothes and curtains, but nicotine is also a powerful stimulant. It causes the release of epinephrine (adrenaline) in the body. The effect is arousal — increased heart rate and a heightened state of awareness. If *you're* the smoker, give up. If you've tried and failed, then at least refrain from smoking before bedtime to avoid its stimulating effects. If your partner is a smoker, get them to do their smoking somewhere else.

Finally, if you can possibly avoid it, don't have a television in the bedroom. In your mind, the bedroom should be associated with sex, relaxation and everything to do with sleep.

Diet

'Breakfast like a king, lunch like a prince and dine like a pauper' goes the old wives' tale, and it seems there's a lot of common sense in this. Inappropriate eating habits can interfere with sleep. Overeating is considered an even greater cause of sleep deprivation than the other extreme — dieting. Boring as the message may seem, moderation is the key.

In general, it is better to eat lightly before going to bed, because the body will not have an opportunity to metabolise a heavy meal properly during sleep. As a result, indigestion may ensue. In the process, you may suffer sufficient discomfort to wake you, or you may have to put up with shallow sleep and bad dreams, from which you waken too easily.

Confine your eating to carbohydrates, such as pasta, muffins and bread, and light snacks such as low-fat milk, yoghurt, cheese, crackers and fruit, or other foods that you can digest easily. Milk contains tryptophan, an amino acid with sleep-inducing properties, so milky foods can be quite beneficial. Milk also contains calcium, which is widely regarded as a muscle relaxant. Fats take several hours to empty from the stomach, so try to stick to low-fat products.

If you are dieting or watching your weight very carefully, forget what you have heard about eliminating high carbohydrate foods such as pasta, wholemeal bread and brown rice from your weight loss regime. Despite the various dieting myths that abound, these foods are low in fat and an excellent source of nutrients. In this respect, they are an important component in the diet of someone seeking good-quality sleep.

A plate of porridge and milk is considered a good sleep inducing combination. Some peptic ulcer sufferers in particular — who often wake up with gnawing hunger pains — report that it has a soothing effect. It is, of course, also very nutritious.

As discussed before, caffeine in all its manifestations taken within four to six hours before retiring to bed is a no-no for people with sleeping difficulties. Most doctors also agree that alcohol in anything other than very small quantities can have a major impact on sleep quality. The specific recommendations on alcohol consumption are set out on pages 19–20. In terms of consuming other liquids, the advice is to keep the quantity down; otherwise, the desire to pass urine will wake you up. This is a particular problem for older people.

Vitamin deficiency may cause sleep disturbance. Some doctors therefore recommend increasing your dietary intake of vitamins C, B1 and zinc, and reducing vitamin A, if you are already taking that as a supplement.

Exercise

It is not possible to write anything meaningful on the subject of good sleep practice without referring to the importance of exercise in your daily routine. The simple rule is — if you possibly can — to exercise, exercise, exercise. People who take vigorous exercise during the day burn up so much energy that, come night time, they will benefit from an energy deficit. And sleep more easily.

In terms of sleep-inducing activity, exercise for leg and arm muscles is best. If you don't play sports — or have another type of formal exercise regime — and want to do something straightforward, try walking for about thirty minutes a day, *at least* four times a week.

If you would like a more structured activity, you might consider three forty-minute sessions of yoga, stretching exercises, t'ai chi or swimming. It's never too late to start one or more of the gentle fitness/relaxation techniques. See below for information on how yoga can help you win the battle for sleep. Research studies have shown that older people who begin a gentle exercise routine after a long period of inactivity fall asleep quicker, and sleep about an hour longer, than those who remain sedentary.

Remember not to attempt strenuous exercise or sports in the hours before bedtime, because that will stimulate the body — the opposite of what you wish to achieve. The other point about late-evening exercise is that it will almost certainly raise body temperature. A high body temperature is *not* conducive to sleep. (Incidentally, that is one of the reasons why a warm bath at night is preferable to a hot bath.)

Exercise also helps the immune system to function more effectively, thereby reducing your susceptibility to colds and other respiratory illnesses, which can interfere with sleep quality. Lack of exercise, on the other hand, may be a factor in sleep problems. One theory is that many insomniacs don't take enough exercise and therefore go to bed with alert bodies, as it were. And so sleep eludes them.

Yoga and Sleep

Meditation is not for him who eats too much. Not for him who eats not at all. Not for him who is overmuch addicted to sleep, or for him who is always awake. But for him who regulates his food and recreation, who is balanced in sleeping, in action and in waking, it shall dispel all unhappiness.

Thus goes a quotation in the ancient Indian book, *The Bhagavad Gita*, written thousands of years ago about the practice of yoga, itself at least five thousand years old. 'Dispel all unhappiness' is a big claim, but it is certainly hard not to be enthusiastic about yoga and the role it can play in promoting general well-being. It can also fix some of the psychological and physiological causes of sleep disturbance.

Yoga is almost the perfect antidote to the worst excesses of modern life. If you lead a typical, late-twentieth-century lifestyle, of relative physical inactivity combined with periods of stress/overload, yoga is an ideal way to achieve deep relaxation, awareness and fitness — without ever getting out of breath. Also on the plus side, it is not as time consuming as other exercise regimes. A single one-and-a-half-hour class a week is sufficient to keep you in gear.

Its other great appeal is that it is as accessible and appropriate for eight- and eighty-year-olds as it is for competitive cyclists, older people with arthritis and harassed business executives. According to Linda Southgate, who has been teaching yoga for sixteen years, anyone can do it:

My pupils have included a double amputee in a wheelchair; drop-out adolescents on a rehabilitation/re-education programme; stressed out exam students and their even more stressed out teachers; postmen suffering from migraine; and young mothers needing time to themselves. There are 80,000 yoga movements in all, but we only use about twenty or thirty in a normal yoga class. I would preclude certain postures for people with high blood pressure or ulcers; and some would be modified for women at certain stages of pregnancy, or people with back pain, but that's about it as far as contra-indications go.

The beauty of yoga is that it uses very slow, gentle movements to exercise every part of the body. It works by releasing energy and removing tension. It takes the body through its full range of movements, thus promoting health and energy. It particularly focuses on the spine, which houses the central nervous system, and that is one of the reasons why yoga is especially good for helping a range of nervous conditions such as stress, anxiety and tension.

It gives you the most incredible feeling of being able to cope. Yoga's effects spill over into the rest of your life, and so cannot but help sleep problems. They say twenty minutes of yoga relaxation is the equivalent of four hours sleep, and in fact people who practise it report needing less sleep.

However, the sleep well/yoga connection isn't universal. Forty-six-year-old Sally, who has been practising yoga for twenty years, is currently menopausal and is experiencing the kind of sleep disturbance very common at that time of life. She wakes every night at least once, and cannot get back to sleep for an hour or more.

Regular practising of yoga doesn't help Sally sleep, but unlike other women in this situation, she doesn't panic about the lack of sleep. She refuses to take medication or other sleep remedies, and says yoga has taught her not to fret and to regard these nightly waking periods as a bonus.

Whereas yoga cannot help overcome that particular aspect of menopausal sleeplessness for Sally, it does, according to Linda Southgate, have a positive impact on some of the other organic causes of sleep disturbance, including:

◆ anxiety
◆ backache
◆ grief
◆ high blood pressure

◆ menstruation

◆ pain from injury

◆ pregnancy

◆ respiratory problems such as asthma, hay fever and bronchitis

◆ stress

◆ stress-related irritable bowel syndrome

◆ tension

◆ tinnitus

◆ ulcers.

One of the beauties of yoga is that some of the asanas — as the movements are called — can be done almost anywhere, such as at home, in the office or while commuting.

Although it can be strenuous, everyone exercises at their own pace. Aerobics it is not, although from an exercise point of view, it can help achieve weight loss, change of body shape and a good level of fitness. It is not a quick fix, however, so if you have serious sleeping problems, be prepared for the long haul if yoga is the route you've chosen.

That said, many people report sleeping very well after just one class. Even harder to imagine is the fact that others fall asleep on hard wooden floors *during* classes, surrounded by up to eighteen other yoga practitioners — such is the level of relaxation they achieve while in the savasana position.

Many people attend yoga classes for decades, and some continue well into their eighties. While it is possible to learn the technique from a book, attending a class really is the optimum. Classes are often mixed: age, gender, ability or lack of experience do not preclude participation.

Each class lasts about one and a half hours, of which about half an hour is devoted to deep relaxation. Much of that time is focused on breathing techniques to calm the mind. These same techniques can later be applied to stress situations, or times when sleep is proving elusive.

Case Studies

To show the positive benefits of yoga, I am including three case studies. To ensure confidentiality, the names of the people have been changed.

Case Study 1
Andrew

Sixteen-year-old Andrew was sent to Linda Southgate by his GP, who was reluctant to prescribe drugs for the boy's anxiety.

Although academically gifted and doing well at school, Andrew still had difficulty coping with daily life, due to his anxious nature. When he started yoga classes, he was rigid with tension, quite withdrawn and often near to tears.

After two to three months, both his physical appearance and his overall outlook changed. Although working very hard and still worrying about the outcome of his forthcoming exams, Andrew felt better able to cope with whatever the final results might be. He plans to continue with yoga in the future.

Case Study 2
Jocelyn

Jocelyn, who is twenty-nine, took up yoga in desperation after a miscarriage was followed by her husband developing long-term clinical depression. A full-time mother with two children aged three and six, she described her life as very stressful. To compound this, she took no exercise and generally felt at the end of her tether. She also reported difficulties in sleeping.

After a few months of attending yoga classes, Jocelyn's self-esteem had improved. She started managing her children better, and was able to cope with her husband's depression by becoming less involved in his problems. She became more aware of her own needs, and in the process her tension and rigid appearance disappeared. Her sleeping problems, which have not returned since, improved greatly. She is continuing with her yoga class routine for the moment.

Case Study 3
Martha

Martha, aged forty-seven, is a former nurse who has had multiple sclerosis since she was twenty-two. She's been paralysed from the waist down and wheelchair bound for four years, during which time she's been completely inactive. One of the side effects of her condition is that she sleeps at least twelve hours out of twenty-four, on and off.

Recently, Linda Southgate has started to do simple yoga postures with her, which Martha finds re-energising. She says she doesn't need as much sleep now. Her self-esteem is improving, and she finds that little by little she's accomplishing a few more tasks every day.

CHAPTER 5

Getting Help

If your sleeping problem has persisted for more than two weeks, your first port of call should be your GP. Because insomnia and sleep disorders are merely a symptom of an underlying cause and not a disease in themselves, establishing the cause is where your doctor will most likely focus his or her efforts initially. If the cause is one of the common illnesses listed in Chapter 3, then clearly it's important to have those addressed first.

If the cause cannot be identified immediately, a psycho-active drug may be prescribed as a temporary, stress-relieving measure. This might be either an anti-depressant or a sleeping pill. You could expect anti-depressants — which have a sleep inducing side-effect — to work for months, but the maximum effectiveness period for sleeping pills tends to be weeks rather than months. So, while they have an important role to play in helping people with sleeping disorders, sleeping pills are not for the long haul.

If your sleeping problems have not been caused by a particular illness, then it may be necessary to refer you to a psychologist, a psychiatrist or a sleep clinic (although the last tends to be fairly rare).

A GP's Perspective

Most people who complain of chronic sleeping problems will sooner or later end up in a GP's surgery looking for sleep-ing pills. The majority of them are probably suffering from depression or some other underlying anxiety-related problem, but don't, won't or can't admit it.

Dr Tiernan Murray, a doctor with a busy practice, who also runs continuing medical education courses for GPs, has strong views on this subject. He says:

Selling depression is a GP's most difficult task. Usually, we can see it, but the patient won't accept it. This prejudice is probably the single biggest reason why patients demand, and end up taking, sleeping tablets that don't work. Not only are they taking the wrong medication for *their* situation, they are also masking and postponing effective treatment for the real problem.

A typical scenario is a long-term non-sleeper, who presents looking for sleeping pills. They try several that don't work. The reason they don't work is that their real problem is an accumulation of anxiety, tipping over into depression. But they won't entertain the idea of going on anti-depressants, because that has overtones of moral weakness.

One of the realities of life we have to face as GPs is that the people who most benefit from taking sleeping pills only represent a small percentage of those who come looking for help. Those for whom hypnotics (sleeping pills) are actually designed have no history of drug or alcohol abuse; no history of chronic psychiatric illness; and are only having temporary anxiety problems as a result of something like the break-up of a relationship, recent bereavement, work-related stress, job loss or some other short-term, but none the less major, life event trauma/upheaval.

Sleeping tablets can have a useful role to play as a short-term solution, in bridging the gap until the problem causing poor sleep in the first instance is dealt with. Very often, a course of anti-depressants, counselling/psycho-logical help, or some appropriate lifestyle change is the optimum route; but in the meantime, chronic sleep deprivation may leave you incapable of thinking clearly or functioning physically. Unfortunately, without fire brigade help in the form of medication, you may not have either the energy, the will, or the ability to address the under-lying problems anyway.

Counselling

Authorities vary in their opinion on the role of counselling in sleep disorders. Ideally, all sufferers should attend for coun-selling, if only for a short period of time, to gain help in tackling underlying psychological problems, or adjustment reactions.

Counselling should be actively considered by those who:

♦ are not ideal candidates for hypnotics
♦ do not quickly respond to short-term hypnotics
♦ present with depression, and respond to treatment, but are keen to explore the underlying problems that may have led to the depression.

According to Dr Murray, counselling as a therapy forms an ideal model of medical care, because we should always consider non-drug treatment before drug treatments. We should value therapies that have long-term preventive value, rather than short-term 'ambulance treatment'. And, finally, we should encourage treatments that empower people to overcome their own problems.

Don't Keep Taking the Tablets

If you are about to start taking sleeping pills, there is a number of simple facts you should be aware of.

There is no such thing as an ideal sleeping pill. The same medication can create completely different reactions in different people. In addition, even though they may be described as, say, six-hour action (i.e. gives you six hours' sleep), that may manifest itself as three hours in one individual and ten in another, depending on age and existing medical conditions.

As already emphasised, they are only ever a short-term solution — maybe for as little as three weeks, depending on the individual and the frequency with which they're taken. If they are taken nightly, sleeping tablets are more likely to become ineffective. Because they can be both psychologically and physically addictive, getting people off them is difficult, so generally it's best not to get started unless you fit in to Dr Murray's ideal candidate category.

Some sleeping pills linger on in the system for up to twenty-four hours, and may affect psycho-motor functions required when operating machinery or driving. The effect on short-term memory can be terrible.

Psycho-active drugs: the chemical family

In the sleeping problems/depression area, the pharmaceutical market has been dominated by two major groups of drugs: benzodiazepines and tricyclics. Increasingly, a newer group of anti-depressants, the SSRIs, are being used.

Barbiturates used to be the third category, but these days they are a controlled drug, like morphine. They are no longer prescribed by GPs and psychiatrists as a matter of course. Their two distinguishing features are that they are highly addictive, and they can kill if a patient overdoses on them. Where they are prescribed, it is usually because a patient has been hooked on them for some time, and it's proving difficult — if not impossible — to wean them off.

Although they have some disadvantages, benzodiazepines, on the other hand, are safe in the sense that it's difficult to overdose on them. If you swallow twenty tablets, you'll probably just sleep for two days without any long-term side effects. Mixing them with alcohol, though, can be very dangerous.

There are numerous brands of benzodiazepines. At the time of writing, there are at least fifteen different ones on the market; they are divided into two categories: hypnotics and anxiolytics.

Hypnotics, in turn, divide into two types: short-acting, which wear off quickly; and long-acting, which keep you asleep throughout the night, but may have a side effect of day-time drowsiness. Hypnotics are sedative — they make you sleepy, so by definition they are sleeping pills.

The second group (anxiolytics) don't make you sleepy, and they function as day-time relaxers. They work by breaking up anxiety and sometimes people use them to aid sleep. The advantage is that this type of benzodiazepine does not result in drowsiness, or a hangover feeling, the next day.

Apart from the benzodiazepine tranquillisers and hypnotics, other psychiatric drugs such as anti-depressants affect sleep — for example, tricyclic anti-depressants. These drugs are primarily anti-depressants, but one of their other effects is to promote sleep. One reason people may have resistance to tricyclic anti-depressants, however, is that these drugs tend to have a lot of side-effects. These range from dry mouth, intermittent blurred vision, daytime drowsiness, slow reflexes (for about the first two weeks of treatment), to constipation and urinary problems (in men with prostate trouble). These are rough guidelines, however, because individual reactions vary enormously: no reaction from people on whacking doses, to debilitating reactions from those on tiny doses.

The GP's Dilemma

So, are GPs being irresponsible in prescribing hypnotics, when they should in fact be prescribing anti-depressants?

The answer, of course, is 'no'. The fault usually lies elsewhere, and the dimensions of the prescribing problem are very complex. Patients may present with depression, but no sleep disturbance, or vice versa. They may have depression and chronic sleep disturbance, in which case an anti-depressant on its own will take too long to have an effect. They may have chronic long-term anxiety, but are not depressed, in which case they may wish to take anxiolytics, but shouldn't. (Once on them, they may never want to come off!)

GPs have to battle with everything — patient expectations, lack of knowledge and awareness of depression and its origins, and patients masking or hiding anxiety problems. Then there is the area of patients having to cope with complex, long-term and intractable social and domestic problems. In extreme situations, retreating into a pharmacological haze may be their only means of survival — however undesirable that is, and however reluctant their GP may be to prescribe anxiolytics long term.

When presented with a crisis situation, most GPs are up against a critical time factor. Sleeping pills start to take effect thirty minutes after entering the body. Anti-depressants require about *two weeks* to take full effect. Therefore, some patients may need a combination of both initially. To further complicate the prescribing problem, the newer SSRI group of anti-depressants are stimulating and may increase sleeping problems. The most important thing of all about taking any sleeping pills is that a patient knows from the outset that they are only for a limited period.

A GP may feel certain that a patient's sleeping difficulties are caused by depression. Until such time as they admit it and recognise the symptoms, however, they may neither agree to take anti-depressants, nor submit to the time-consuming (and sometimes expensive) process of counselling, or go about tackling their problems in another way.

By far the most common category of patient with a sleeping problem is someone with chronic anxiety. For this type of patient, hypnotics are against the rules, because their problem is long-term. They will develop tolerance to hypnotics within a few weeks. They may even become physically or psychologically addicted. What this patient needs is an anti-depressant. Not only will it help with day-to-day living, but sleep will improve because of its sedative effect, and relaxation will also follow.

Patients can stay on anti-depressants for months, even years, without any ill effect. Meantime, however, their underlying lifestyle problems will remain untreated, so from a GP's point of view, there are both philosophical and psychological reasons for not favouring prescriptions longer than three to twelve months.

Getting the Best Results from Sleeping Pills

In order to get the best results from sleeping pills, Dr Tiernan Murray recommends taking one every night for the first week. Then begin to take just a few a week. For example, if you have had two bad nights, take one the following night. After that, maintain this irregular pattern for a maximum of about three weeks, or as long as the temporary crisis lasts.

Do I Have Depression?

Anti-depressants really work, and Dr Murray adds: 'Psychiatrists commonly express the view that GPs prescribe anti-depressants too infrequently, at too small a dose, for too short a period. Many GPs would agree, but plead practical difficulties.'

Part of the problem lies with patients themselves, who object to the labelling anti-depressants confer on them, and so may resist that kind of prescription. The kind of anti-drug culture (relatively speaking) that pervades society in Ireland

and the UK is also partly responsible for this resistance to anti-depressants. (Consumption of drugs in both countries is at the bottom of the Western Europe league table, according to Dr Murray.)

Generating greater public awareness of depression and its key signs is an ongoing battle. Dr Murray says that the single most useful piece of literature in his waiting room is a poster highlighting the common signs of depression. Very often, patients who might have planned to ask for sleeping pills change their mind by the time they've made it into the surgery. Prior to reading the poster, the idea that they were suffering from depression might never have entered their minds, but by the time they have answered 'yes' to at least four of the questions listed, they will already have begun the process of diagnosing the cause of their current sleeping difficulties. In this situation, everyone wins.

The Depression Checklist

If you have had *four or more* of the following symptoms for more than two weeks, you probably have depression and should consult your GP for help.

1 Are you feeling persistently sad or anxious, or do you have an empty feeling?
2 Are you tired or slowed down, despite rest?
3 Have you lost interest in food, sex, work?
4 Are you wakening during the night, or too early in the morning, or having trouble getting to sleep?
5 Have you lost (without dieting) or gained weight?
6 Are you having difficulty thinking, remembering or making decisions?
7 Are you feeling guilty or worthless?
8 Have you been having thoughts of death or suicide?
9 Do you have aches or pains without a physical cause?

Usually — but not always — problems such as difficulty getting off to sleep, early morning waking or oversleeping (say nine/ten hours or more), will go hand in hand with depression. It is, however, possible to be severely depressed and not have any of these particular sleeping problems.

Dr Murray's Case Studies

Case Study 1
Amanda

Amanda is thirty years old and single. She works as a nurse, and moved home from abroad to look after her dying mother. Two weeks after her mother's death, she asked for sleeping pills. Contributing factors clearly included grief over her mother's death; a combination of sleep disturbance and deprivation over a six-week period; and coping with living temporarily in a new environment.

On the plus side, Amanda had never taken hypnotics before, was psychologically well, and had no past history of sleep disturbance.

Her treatment consisted of support from her GP; encouragement to vent her feelings; information on the normal grieving process; advice to attend support groups, including a hospice post-bereavement course; and a prescription for a two- to three-week course of hypnotics.

The outcome was extremely successful: a quick return to her normal sleeping pattern. Amanda went back to her job in the UK shortly afterwards, and sent Dr Murray a postcard four weeks later saying all was well and thanks!

Case Study 2
Sally

Sally is forty-six, married and a full-time mother. She has suffered from a long history of difficulty sleeping. She could not get to sleep, and lay in bed with the problems of the day running through her head. If she did get to sleep, she woke up again, sometimes because of her husband's snoring or her teenage sons returning home. She then found it impossible to return to sleep, and was worn out as a result.

On close questioning by her GP, there were no definite symptoms of depression, and she in any case strongly denied that possibility. Sally did, however, admit to having had headaches for years (probably from tension); to being tense quite often; and to having a perfectionist personality. She also added that she got aching shoulders and jaws due to muscle tension.

Very reluctantly, she agreed to take a tricyclic for two weeks. After that, she reported that she was sleeping much better and felt more relaxed the next day. Her headaches disappeared.

Dr Murray repeated the prescription for a further four weeks. After a total of six weeks on medication, she reported feeling great: 'I haven't felt so well in years. Minor problems don't bother me any more, and my tiredness has lessened greatly.'

After three months, Sally still reported feeling terrific and asked if she could stay on the pills. Dr Murray agreed. He adds:

Is she on them for life? Probably not. After about one year, she may well come off them without the symptoms returning. However, ideally, during that time, she should attend a psychologist for some advice on non-drug methods of relaxation/stress avoidance, or more involved work on the background factors that led to the problems in the first place.

Case Study 3
Cilla

Sixty-three-year-old Cilla is the active wife of a retired businessman. She is very dedicated to her family and to charity work.

Having attended Dr Murray's surgery regularly for blood pressure and HRT (hormone replacement therapy), she on one occasion said: 'I'm having terrible trouble sleeping. I took a few of my husband's sleepers. They initially seemed good, but now they only give me three hours' sleep. Can you give me a better one?' In the limited time available on that occasion, her GP probed for evidence of anxiety or depression, but met with great resistance.

Dr Murray takes up the story:

Reluctantly, I prescribed a different hypnotic, but without benefit to the patient, who now began to manifest with a variety of non-specific physical symptoms and morbid fear of illness. A battery of hospital tests and x-rays proved normal.

Then, the penny finally dropped. More detailed discussion revealed the common picture of the self-sacrificing mother, still very involved in helping her children, their spouses and their own children. Over-involved in charity work, where she felt she had made herself indispensable; worried about her husband's recent ill health, but unable to fully discuss her own problems with him. The picture of increasing anxiety, decreasing coping ability and descent into depression was now very evident.

I started her on SSRIs. Due to the relatively slow onset of action, she needed great support from me through the first two weeks. Gradually, she began to improve, and at six weeks was back to her old self. She will need to stay on medication for three to twelve months. However, much will depend on how she handles the critical factors in her life. Factors such as learning how to say 'no' to the charity; detaching from over-involvement in family; selecting new activities for herself chosen on an entirely selfish basis (i.e. for herself alone, not for others); and planning anew, with her husband, how they will shape and enjoy their post-retirement life together.

If she accomplishes these aims, she can look forward with confidence to a comfortable life without medication. If not, she risks requiring long-term medication (best avoided if possible), or relapsing into depression as she goes on and off medication during the coming years.

Case Study 4
Katie

Katie is a frail but broadly healthy seventy-two-year-old. She had only recently moved into the area and so joined Dr Murray's practice. She was on medication and attended for a repeat prescription. Specifically, she needed a repeat for a well-known hypnotic, which she had taken every night for six years since the death of her husband. She insisted that she could not sleep without it, and described how she hated the thought of lying awake at night, fearful of every noise.

Dr Murray gently broached the area of side-effects — memory impairment; poor reflexes; risk of falls and resultant fractures (falls while getting up to go to the toilet during the night, or during the day); risk of car accidents (decreased reflexes); and addictive properties. Katie was having none of this: 'I'm grand, doctor. The tablets suit me and if I'm addicted at seventy-two, so what?'

The GP prescribed her a hypnotic, and continues to do so to this day. Dr Murray notes that this is one of the commoner scenarios: 'It is very difficult for a GP to refuse a perceived need for a harmless little helper. If Katie came off the hypnotic, she would eventually sleep just as well without it. However, she simply was not interested in trying.'

Many GPs are sympathetic to such patients, and do not feel their requests are unreasonable. Life can be difficult, and in an ideal world, nobody would need any medication. As Dr Murray says: 'We have to live in the world as it exists, with all its vicissitudes, and try to use pharmacology as wisely as possible to draw on its many obvious benefits.'

Coming Off Sleeping Pills

If you have been on sleeping pills for some time, going cold turkey is a very bad idea. Nobody should try and wean themselves off medication without the advice of a doctor. Depending on whether you are on a combination of, say, tranquillisers and hypnotics, Dr Catherine Crowe's advice is to come off them *one at a time*. (Individual cases will dictate which comes first in the weaning-off sequence.)

Dr Crowe notes:

Generally, I would not reduce at a rate greater than one single dose per week, and for most people it would be even slower than that. Say, for instance, someone is taking 30 mg of Dalmane, which comes in 15 mg and 30 mg capsules; then they would reduce their nightly dose to 15 mg for one to four weeks, and then stop. Or they might take half a Dalmane 15 mg capsule for a further few weeks before completely stopping.

The time taken to reduce medication depends on type, dose and length of hypnotic consumption (months or years), as well as individual factors. Not everyone will stick with the full process, but even partial reduction is still an achievement. Rebound insomnia tends to occur in short-acting hypnotics, but is less of a problem with the longer-acting ones. That said, most people should expect some difficulty for a week or two after coming off them, and it could be months before sleep readjusts to a level they are really happy with.

Anyone coming off sleeping pills can help themselves by doing yoga, relaxation therapy or even acupuncture. I would never favour leaving a patient bereft of support.

CHAPTER 6

Sleep Clinics

According to Dr Catherine Crowe, typically patients are referred to her clinic by a GP for investigation and treatment for a variety of problems. These include:

◆ snoring/sleep apnoea: 60%
◆ insomnia: 20%
◆ excessive day-time sleepiness, including narcolepsy: 15%
◆ miscellaneous — including nightmares, sleep walking, restless legs syndrome and other rarer conditions: 5%.

Despite the complexity surrounding sleep, in almost all cases Dr Crowe and her team can arrive at a diagnosis of the source of the problem fairly quickly. Treatments, surprisingly, are also relatively straightforward.

How are Sleep Disorders Investigated?
Polysomnography

In the case of severe snoring or suspected sleep apnoea, the investigation is often initiated by a distracted partner whose own sleep is being impaired. Their complaints can start a process which may begin with consulting a GP, and end with a sleep disorders specialist, or a sleep clinic, for more detailed diagnosis and treatment.

Following a consultation with the sleep disorders specialist, the patient may be booked into a sleep clinic for one night's observation and tests to confirm diagnosis and the severity of the condition.

During the afternoon — or prior to retiring at their normal bedtime — a technician attaches electrodes (little sensors) to various parts of the body to record brain waves continuously, muscle activity, eye movements and heart rhythm. The patient will also be given a device to wear around the waist and chest to record respiratory effort. A sensor may also be attached to a leg to check for kicks.

In the case of snoring/sleep apnoea patients, they will also have a small moustache-like sensor between the nose and mouth to measure airflow. Finally, a clip will be placed on one finger tip to measure oxygen levels. Hypersomnia patients generally follow the same procedure as sleep apnoea patients. The procedure is usually the same for insomnia patients, although the moustache and oxygen clip may be left off.

This sleep measurement equipment sounds cumbersome, but surprisingly it is neither particularly intrusive nor uncomfortable. A reasonable night's sleep generally ensues, thereby giving the sleep disorders specialist an overview of the patient's sleep, breathing and heart function. This can be particularly revealing in the case of insomnia sufferers, who are often convinced that they sleep a great deal less than they actually do. The sleep clinic can produce scientific and reassuring evidence to the contrary.

Multiple Sleep Latency Test — Maintenance of Wakefulness Test

These are nap tests carried out during the day, following a full night's recording, and are carried out on excessively sleepy patients. They help evaluate the type and severity of the sleepiness.

The maintenance of wakefulness test is useful where there is a doubt about a patient's capacity to drive or supervise machinery.

Advances in Technology

Until fairly recently, sleep clinic recordings involved a tedious, time-consuming process, requiring a technician to be present to monitor both patients and equipment throughout the night. The different measurements were then printed out on vast quantities of paper.

More recent technology still measures eight hours of complex and enormously varied reactions. The difference is that the information is gathered electronically. This has several advantages. Apart from saving on paper, it also means that it's no longer necessary to have a technician hovering around all night — an aspect of the process some patients used to find a bit off-putting.

The new sleep clinic process is also less expensive than heretofore, since technicians no longer have to be paid to work through the night. They are free to leave once the equipment has been set up properly. After that, such supervision as is necessary can easily be carried out by nursing staff on duty at the hospital looking after non-sleep clinic patients on the ward or, in exceptional cases, in the intensive care unit.

The next day, the patient returns home. On the same day — or soon after — the sleep disorders specialist, or trained technician, scores the entire night's polysomnography recording with the aid of the computer. Diagnosis tends to be both swift and accurate — particularly if sleep apnoea or narcolepsy is the source of the problem.

Sleep Apnoea Treatment

If moderate to severe sleep apnoea is diagnosed, the patient will be asked to return to the clinic for two or three nights, where he will be adapted to nasal CPAP (pronounced *see-pap*). This would normally entail at least one night's polysomnography, to ensure that the correct pressure is being used. The patient is also taught to use the CPAP breathing apparatus when he is at home.

When they are discharged from hospital, patients are instructed to use the apparatus all night, every night. Side effects from CPAP are frequent, although minor, initially. These include mask leaks and skin problems caused by the mask. If excessive dryness of the nasal passages — or the opposite, excessive sneezing and runny nose — occur during the day, a humidifier may be needed. This can be added quite simply to the machine.

Most of the problems can be dealt with easily, and after the first few weeks the majority of patients have minimum problems. Treatment is successful in the majority of cases and most patients feel greatly improved.

However, Dr Crowe says that relationship problems are common in couples where one partner has sleep apnoea. Apart from the aggravation of chronic snoring, there are other factors including depression, irritability, memory loss, intellectual deterioration and impotence in men, combined with excessive sleepiness during the day, which may be severe.

In many cases, the 'well' half of the partnership is effectively living with someone who is physically present, but psychologically absent. Over a period of months or years, they may have either developed a life of their own outside the marriage, or simply got accustomed to living with a very absent partner. Following the treatment, however, they may end up with a partner who now has a quite different personality and behaviour pattern — mended certainly, but totally unlike what they may have been used to for months, or years, on end. That kind of dramatic change can put a relationship under strain, so Dr Crowe says that patients are carefully counselled about what to expect.

Children may also have difficulty coming to terms with a father who was previously very passive and didn't take much notice of them. Suddenly, they are confronted with someone who may be taking a keen interest in what they're doing or *not* doing. It's not that the sleep apnoea patient's behaviour is worse — it's just that it's *changed* — and dramatic change can be bewildering.

Chronotherapy

Chronotherapy is the name given to one of the processes for treating insomniacs. Translated into lay terminology, this is the method by which a wonky biological clock is reset.

This treatment tends to be most successful for people with so-called night owl syndrome; those who have got into the bad habit of going to bed later and later each night and who, as a consequence, tend to sleep later and later each day, until they are completely out of sync with the world around them. This kind of insomnia is quite common among teenagers and students (particularly if they have the kind of lectures schedule that doesn't require them to appear in class early every morning). If a regular schedule of early rising every day of the week for several weeks does not work, chronotherapy might help.

Chronotherapy is a simple process. The treatment rule of thumb is to get patients to advance their sleep schedule by three hours every night, until after about eight consecutive nights, they get back to where they want to be. According to Dr Crowe, it is absolutely essential that they maintain a regular schedule after that. They simply must get up at the same time *every* day. If they don't, they could be subjecting their bodies and their biological clocks to the equivalent of making a trip from London to New York every weekend. Not to be recommended.

A note of caution: although straightforward, chronotherapy is *not* a DIY method of treating insomnia. It is best carried out under the direction of a sleep disorders specialist, or a GP.

Light Therapy

The reason why our bodies re-synchronise on a daily basis is due to light. It works by reinforcing quite strongly the natural night and day alternation. As a result, in people who have a tendency to sleep late, light then gives a very clear signal that night is over.

Light therapy is, essentially, a sleep time regulator. It stimulates the brain to push back the time of sleep. Like chronotherapy, it is best carried out under the direction of a sleep disorders specialist, or GP. It is most beneficial for the treatment of delayed or advanced phase syndrome. It works particularly well for people who have developed a tendency to wake up late.

The treatment process is extremely straightforward. The patient either rents or buys a special light box which emits very strong light — 10,000 lux. (To put that figure into perspective, the light in an average bedroom in Dublin, Edinburgh or London on a typical afternoon in early November would be about 500 lux.)

For two weeks, for about one hour first thing each morning, the patient sits in a room, exposed to the light emitted from the box. The box can be placed on the breakfast table, or any other area where the morning ritual is being carried out. Once the desired rhythm is achieved, patients need to maintain a very regular schedule. Otherwise, they will slip back into very bad habits again.

CHAPTER 7

Autogenic Training, Homeopathy and Acupuncture

What is Autogenic Training?

Autogenic training is sometimes confused with meditation, from which it differs by inducing specific normalising processes in the body-mind, rather than trying to transcend them, as in meditation.

Essentially, it is a form of self-hypnosis, used to bring about profound relaxation and relief from the negative effects of stress. 'Autogenic' means generated from within, and the technique consists of a series of simple, easily learned mental exercises which allow the mind to calm itself by switching off the body's stress system. It's easy to do and, once learned, almost impossible to forget — a bit like riding a bicycle.

Although it has been taught in many European countries, North America and the Far East for decades, it is relatively new to the UK and Ireland. It was first introduced here in the late 1970s, and the total number of trainers is still under a hundred. This is possibly due to the stringent requirements for acceptance, coupled with a relatively long training period — three years part time — on top of existing training and qualifications in medicine, nursing, counselling or psychology.

Dr Alice Greene, a Harley Street homeopathic doctor, started her training in autogenics in the mid 1980s, while she was a practising GP. Now Vice-Chairwoman of the British

Association for Autogenic Training and Therapy (BAFATT), she says it can be used to support and enhance progress in other therapies, or provide a non-drug approach for many problems.

Who Is Autogenic Training For?

It isn't necessary to be ill, stressed or have sleeping problems to benefit from autogenic training. Many people use it to improve efficiency by sharpening their awareness and discernment. Others use it to mobilise creativity, or facilitate personal growth and inner development. Olympic athletes have used it successfully to improve their performance.

One of the greatest exponents of autogenic training, Dr Hannes Lindemann, used it to get across the Atlantic single-handedly in a boat, when he was suffering from exhaustion and frostbite. American and Russian astronauts have been taught it to aid relaxation and physiological normalisation. Airline pilots and cabin crews use it to cope with sleep difficulties caused by jet lag, and to keep them relaxed and alert. Management training organisations offer it to high-powered business executives to help reduce their stress levels.

Aside from those with sleep disorders, type A personalities — typically over-stretched, ambitious, stressed, competitive, high-achieving, impatient and restless — tend to benefit most. It brings about a profound shift in their personalities. Their adrenalised state disappears. Autogenics allows them to relax, and sleep follows. People in the caring professions, such as nurses, doctors, ambulance drivers, policemen and social workers, who can easily become emotionally exhausted and overwhelmed, also benefit.

One UK National Health Service hospital provides autogenic training for out-patients suffering from a wide variety of disorders. And some alcoholism treatment specialists encourage patients to practise it. This is because it has been shown to reduce the drop-out rate among those undergoing out-patient treatment and therapy.

As far as the general public is concerned, however, autogenics is still a relatively uncommon practice, despite being one of the most dramatically successful profound relaxation methods around.

Evaluating Your Suitability

Pre-course evaluation is essential to assess a patient's suitability for autogenic training. There are a very few people for whom it's not suitable: people on major tranquillisers; those with psychiatric disorders, but who are not under medical supervision; people with schizophrenia, or psychoses; those suffering with endogenous (coming from within) depression, for which they are on long-term medication. Diabetics who are not under medical supervision are also precluded, because autogenics can bring about a reduction in their need for insulin.

Others precluded are those whose medical history is not available, or who refuse to give it; people with severe chest pain (where there may be an imminent heart attack); and children under five.

Although people with severe endogenous depression are precluded, those with reactive depression may find it very helpful. Likewise, post-heart attack patients find it a very useful rehabilitation therapy. Autogenics is cardio-protective, in that it reduces stress, lowers lipids, increases coronary blood flow and reduces blood pressure and pulse rate.

Autogenics and Sleep Disorders

There are now some 3,000 scientific studies demonstrating the effectiveness of autogenics in the treatment of a wide range of disorders. These include high blood pressure; asthma; irritable bowel syndrome and colitis; arthritis; muscular pain and tension; migraines; bladder disorders; sexual dysfunction; cardiac arrhythmias; angina; mild thyroid disorders; epilepsy; pain relief in childbirth; pre-menstrual tension; digestive disturbances; and sleep problems.

Sleep and anxiety are closely interlinked, and of the many physiological changes reported during the autogenic process, anxiety reduction is a central one. Other areas where autogenics can help include reactive depression; panic attacks; unresolved grief reactions; anxiety disorders and phobias. It can be enormously beneficial to those suffering from post traumatic stress disorder. It can also help — under proper supervision — in the process of weaning people off tranquillisers, hypnotics and anti-depressant drugs.

Studies have shown autogenics to be extremely effective in the treatment of sleep disorders, ranging from difficulty in falling asleep and disrupted sleep (followed by difficulty in falling asleep again), to wakening too early in the morning. In addition, sleep problems which are the side effect of organic diseases (like hypothyroidism, arteriosclerosis, diabetes and hypertension), and insomnia caused by rheumatic, neuralgic or dental pain, also respond well to autogenic training.

Other studies have shown that even in those without sleep disorders, changes in the person's usual sleep pattern occur after training. Dreams are remembered more vividly, and previously anxiety-laden dreams take a more pleasant turn. People report sleeping better and needing less sleep. They fall asleep more quickly, feel more refreshed than usual in the morning, and find it easier to get up. Even your typical morning grouch may change and report feeling joyful first thing!

How Does Autogenics Work?

I will leave it to Dr Alice Greene's own words to describe the process:

Autogenic training is a system of profound relaxation and stress management, that works by re-balancing the autonomic nervous system. This system is divided into two sides. One is the fight-and-flight mechanism of adrenaline arousal; the other is the relaxation, rest, repair, healing and digestive side of the nervous system. When people get over-anxious, they become dominated by the arousal side, and find it very difficult to let go and relax. This creates both physiological and psychological effects.

By undoing the doing and placing the mind and body in the 'at rest' mode, it facilitates deep relaxation and nor-malisation of many physiological processes within the body, such as high heart rate, sweating, blood pressure, breathing rate, and increases gut movement and digestion. It brings about concordance of both sides of the brain to facilitate the off loading of emotional blockages and prob-lems and, in doing so, facilitates even deeper levels of rest. All the time you are doing this, you are *totally aware* — as a passive observer — of the balancing process taking place.

It is often used to wean people off tranquillisers and sleeping pills, but we would recommend they stay on medication while undertaking their course of autogenics. However, when the course begins to bite and they begin to feel more relaxed, they can cut down their tablets in an agreed fashion. And then stay off them permanently.

Dr Greene adds:

Specific sleeping problems apart, in my ten years of teach-ing autogenics, I have had a number of patients who didn't realise they slept badly until they did a course, and then spontaneously reported improved sleep (deeper sleep and more refreshing sleep), as well as an improved sense of well-being.

An autogenic training course takes between eight and ten weeks, with one sixty- to ninety-minute class once a week. Numbers are small — usually six to eight per class. In between, all that's necessary are three ten-minutes-a-day practice sessions, of various exercises and positions. No special clothing or equipment is necessary.

Technically, it is possible to learn autogenics from books, but that is not recommended. A properly qualified trainer is vital. Because transient emotional off loadings are part of the process, it's essential to have a qualified person there to help hold the process and monitor temporary changes to the new level of well-being.

After a while, it can be practised anywhere: in the back of a taxi going around Piccadilly Circus at rush hour; at an office desk; on an aircraft. It's an unobtrusive process, so if discretion is your thing, no one need ever know what you're doing.

In conclusion, autogenics is in that grey zone where it may be a treatment if you have a serious illness. It may be a form of relaxation if you are one of the 'worried well'. That said, it is not *just* a relaxation technique. It has profound physiological and psychological consequences, which move towards healing, but may ameliorate transient periods of disturbance, while the person is getting better. These need to be recognised, attended to and dealt with therapeutically and properly, to bring the person through to a level of self-autonomy and safety.

Demand for autogenic training far exceeds supply at present, but although numbers of trainers are low, their geographical spread is quite good. See Useful Addresses, page 104, for a contact and telephone number to consult in order to find a properly qualified trainer.

Homeopathy

Homeopathy is the medical practice of treating like with like. In other words, you treat an illness with a dilution of a substance that in a healthy person produces similar symptoms to those displayed by the person who is ill. An easier way to understand this concept is to compare it with conventional methods such as vaccination, or the use of controlled radiation to treat cancer, which can itself be caused by radiation.

How Does It Work?

Homeopathy aims to stimulate the body's own healing forces, rather than suppress the symptoms. Medicine is administered in minuscule doses, diluted by factors ranging from several thousandths to many millionths of the original substance. Naturally occurring substances are used: plants, minerals and animal extracts. Because of their great dilution, homeopathic medicines are generally free of side-effects and do not create withdrawal symptoms. They are taken for the least amount of time possible, and they are inexpensive.

Generally, homeopathy works slowly, although with sleeping problems it can be reasonably quick in someone who is otherwise well. It is, therefore, an option well worth considering, although access to a homeopathic doctor may not be as easy as to a GP. Homeopathic remedies, on the other hand, are widely available. For straightforward sleeping problems, self-medication may be appropriate. Where anxiety or depression are the underlying causes, however, first aid won't be enough.

According to Dr Brendan Fitzpatrick, a Dublin-based physician who has worked in the UK, Australia and Thailand and who has a special interest in complementary medicines, homeopathy differs from allopathic medicine in one fundamental way:

The underlying philosophy of this treatment is that every person is different, and so the same medicines, dietary regimes and directives do not apply universally.

Treatments will vary, depending on factors such as other physical symptoms, mental and emotional status and the general susceptibilities and sensitivities of the person concerned.

Dr Fitzpatrick goes on:

As a homeopathic doctor, I would always look at the overall picture, using an extremely detailed questionnaire to assess the person's diet, possible vitamin and mineral deficiency/imbalance and emotional stresses. I would also assess their inherited pre-dispositions to certain illnesses, and the possibility of allergies.

I would always examine their tea/coffee intake. Apart from stimulating the nervous system, tea and coffee displace zinc and magnesium, so in cases where intake is high, I'd recommend calcium, zinc or magnesium to help the nervous system.

Likewise, if someone is suffering from low blood sugar ... and reacts by waking up in the middle of the night feeling uneasy or jittery, I might recommend chromium supplements with an appropriate diet to level out their blood sugar. If restless legs are a cause of insomnia, I would recommend vitamin E or calcium or magnesium for this condition.

These are just some of the possible dietary supplements that may be required. In terms of homeopathic medicines, Dr Fitzpatrick usually works with about six to eight medicines for simple sleep disturbance. Medicine selection depends on the nature of the sleep problem and the person's overall personality.

Homeopathic Medicines for Sleep Disorders

Examples are:

- *arnica* for someone who has insomnia as a result of pressure and mental stress, or who has been bruised by life
- *arsenicum* for jittery, fidgety, restless, perfectionist types
- *argentum nitrosum* for people who have anxiety prior to a forthcoming event, such as an interview, presentation or public performance
- *coffea* (a tiny dilution of the coffee bean) for someone with a racing mind, in overdrive; with restless legs or noise sensitivity
- *ignatia* for someone full of grief, weepy or depressed
- *nux vomica* for irritable types/mentally active
- *phosphorous* for sensitive people prone to nightmares.

In instances where sleeping problems have a psychiatric origin, homeopathy may still have a role, but it is usually a matter of proceeding with caution. Dr Fitzpatrick would not stop a patient taking anti-depressants, for example, until certain they were beginning to improve. He applies the same caution to patients suffering from asthma or arthritis.

In conclusion, he adds:

> I use homeopathy on all my patients but if someone asked me does it work for sleeping problems, I'd say the combined picture of homeopathy plus the right adjustments to diet and supplements would do very well, whereas homeopathy on its own might only get a certain number of people right.

Taking the Medication

The rules in relation to taking homeopathic medications are simple, but quite different from any other regime. They are best taken:

- exclusively on their own
- not within thirty minutes of food
- on a teaspoon, remembering not to handle them at any stage.

You should avoid taking them immediately after eating spicy foods, using strong toothpaste, or tobacco.

Whereas many conventional medications hamper or block the effect of homeopathic ones, you should never — as has been emphasised earlier — go cold turkey on sleeping pills, tranquillisers and related medications without consulting your doctor first.

Acupuncture

The first documented recordings of acupuncture techniques date back more than 3,000 years, while the practice itself is believed to be 4,000 or 5,000 years old. In China, it is still regarded as conventional medicine, whereas in the West it is widely regarded as an alternative therapy. In most European countries, only qualified doctors can practise acupuncture. The UK and Ireland, however, are exceptions to that rule.

Chinese-born Dr Katherine Chan Mullen is a member of the Royal Academy of Medicine in Ireland. She was awarded the honour of Distinguished Doctor in Western and Chinese Medicine at the International Conference on Alternative Medicine held at Southern California University in 1995. Having worked in London and Hong Kong, Dr Chan Mullen today practises as a GP and medical acupuncturist in Dublin.

Dr Chan Mullen believes that the popularity of acupuncture, with both patients and doctors, derives from three main reasons:

- its highly successful results
- its holistic approach
- the fact that treatment doesn't create any side-effects.

Acupuncture and Sleep Disorders

According to Dr Chan Mullen, acupuncture doesn't help all sleeping problems. However, she achieves excellent results with short-term insomnia (of three to six weeks' duration); and with sleeping problems caused by depression, anxiety, recent bereavement, trauma or emotional upset. Dr Chan Mullen says that: 'Insomnia has complicated causes. I select my cases for acupuncture treatment very carefully, and therefore report good success rates. I believe precise diagnosis and good selection are crucial to a successful outcome.'

A large number of patients are still on sleeping pills when they begin treatment with Dr Chan Mullen. After acupuncture treatments, however, they manage to wean themselves off medication gradually. Booster treatments may be necessary to prevent a relapse, though. With insomnia, there is never a quick cure. Patience is an important factor to be borne in mind by both patients and doctors.

Who Can Benefit?

People in most age groups respond well to acupuncture, but young people probably achieve the best results overall. Acupuncture is not very effective for chronic, long-term insomnia — either lifestyle induced, or caused by severe clinical depression. Neither is it effective in situations where patients have been taking sleeping pills for a long time.

Although she also practises conventional medicine, Dr Chan Mullen's advice for someone seeking help with sleep disorders is to look at alternative therapies before resorting to traditional Western medicine. She welcomes the conventional medical establishment's move towards considering alternative therapies first before prescribing sleeping tablets.

According to Dr Chan Mullen, the major benefit of acupuncture over herbal medicine or homeopathy is that whereas these therapies introduce medicine into the body —

albeit natural ones — acupuncture does not. In addition, the effect may be temporary and, once stopped, the body has to readjust. Acupuncture, on the other hand, doesn't introduce anything into the body, and so helps the process of self-healing.

Treatment Regime

Acupuncture is administered during six to eight thirty-minute sessions. These are given at weekly intervals to begin with, reducing to fortnightly sessions after four weeks or so. Repeat sessions may be necessary if sleeping problems return some time later. The difficulty is that insomnia has many causes. For example, if a patient's overall health or lifestyle suddenly changes, follow-up may be required to treat the reactive insomnia derived from the new/aggravating conditions.

Like some other alternative medicines and therapies, acupuncture works fairly slowly. For the first two weeks after their referral to her, Dr Chan Mullen allows patients to stay on sleeping pills. After three or four weeks, however, she gradually reduces the medication. This weaning-off regime does not necessarily apply to anti-depressants. A patient can stay on such medication, if desired, without it interfering with the acupuncture treatment.

CHAPTER 8

Complementary Medicine and Therapies

U ntil recent years, complementary medicine had not been part of traditional Western medical school training. As a result, there has been resistance to non-orthodox, non-allopathic remedies, such as acupuncture, reflexology, aromatherapy, homeopathy and medical herbalism.

Orthodox medical practitioners explain their resistance by stating that most complementary therapies and remedies do not have the backup of sufficient clinical trials data and statistics. They're quite right, of course. By and large, scientific research in this area is fairly thin on the ground. This probably has more to do with market and economic factors than unwillingness on the part of complementary medicine practitioners to submit their therapies to expensive and time-consuming scientific evaluation methods.

Slowly but surely, however, the pattern is changing. Almost half the medical schools in the US now have courses in some of these areas. In Germany, medical students must pass an exam on natural medicine, while in the UK and Ireland, study of this area is still not obligatory and is therefore underdeveloped.

Complementary therapies definitely have a role to play in treating common sleep disorders like insomnia and malsomnia. A word of caution is appropriate here. Because many complementary treatments may involve the release of toxins as part of the healing process, therapists believe these need time to settle down. Therefore, they advise that it is not a good idea to mix more than one type of treatment therapy at a time.

Other cautionary notes include not taking certain treatments while pregnant, and expecting the possibility of feeling quite unwell at some stage during the treatment process. It is also important to advise both your doctor and complementary practitioner if you are using other therapies or medications — in case certain conditions, or medications, are contra-indicated for you.

Finally, finding the right therapy may require a lot of trial and error on your part. Universal rules do not apply in medicine, and individual reactions may vary enormously. The best advice is to seek out the relevant governing body for the particular therapy you favour. See Useful Addresses, page 104, for contact addresses and telephone numbers. Ask for a list of the appropriately qualified therapists in your area. If you can, make the final decision based on a personal recommendation from friends or contacts. If you're still not sure, check out the therapist's premises personally.

Credentials and professionalism matter — so does insurance in case anything goes wrong. Properly qualified practitioners should have cover and, generally speaking, insurance companies will check out qualifications and credentials carefully. Be vigilant, and beware of charlatans or unqualified practitioners.

This chapter will look in some detail at a couple of therapies, herbal medicine and aromatherapy.

Herbal Medicine

Treating symptoms is bad medicine — you should treat the cause, not the symptoms. In some respects, modern medicine has forgotten that, which is where herbalism scores: herbalists treat the whole person.

Dr Desmond Corrigan is Head of the Department of Pharmacognosy (medicinal plant studies) at the School of

Pharmacy, Trinity College Dublin; Chairman of the European Scientific Co-operative on Phytotherapy; former analyst with the Irish Drugs Squad. He is also author of *Herbal Medicine for Sleep and Relaxation.*

Although not a medical practitioner, Dr Corrigan 'would prefer to see people using remedies that don't create more problems than they actually solve. That's where I would be particularly worried about benzodiazepines.' He believes that these drugs should be used to treat insomnia only when it is severe and disabling. He is also convinced that hypnotics should not be prescribed indiscriminately, and that routine prescribing is undesirable: 'Ideally, they should be reserved for short courses in the acutely distressed.'

Dr Corrigan says:

I see a useful role for alternative options such as the various relaxation therapies, as well as reflexology, aromatherapy and herbal remedies in the treatment of *mild* insomnia; in other words insomnia that is not disabling and in situations that don't require benzodiazepines or a similar medication; situations where people still feel they need something to help.

The one most intensively researched and which I would have no hesitation in recommending to anyone is valerian. Even though we still haven't identified which chemicals are responsible for its sedative effect, the evidence still justifies its use. I would not consider it an alternative medicine. Rather, it is mainstream medicine that happens to be a plant, as opposed to a synthetic chemical.

Valerian is widely available in pharmacies and health food stores as an over-the-counter preparation. It's not a particularly dangerous plant and it's not poisonous. It's quite unlike benzodiazepines, which can be very dangerous if taken in overdose with alcohol, or barbiturates which can kill if a patient miscalculates the dose accidentally. (The margin for error there between the medical dose and the fatal dose is very small.)

My top three herbal sedatives/tranquillisers are valerian on its own, or valerian mixed with passiflora or hops. Then, to a lesser extent, I would favour chamomile, lime and motherwort. Hops on its own, in my view, is not really active enough. All these remedies can be bought over the counter and are safe, although I would add the caveat that *no* medicine is entirely safe. These remedies are, however, much safer than benzodiazepines which are both physically and psychologically addictive.

Different brands are available, and in the absence of a pharmacist's advice, consumers should look for a mark stating pharmacopoeial quality to (BP or EP) British/European quality standards. This indicates that the remedies have been reviewed by an expert committee, and that the manufacturer has been inspected to ensure the medications have been produced under pharmaceutical conditions in terms of hygiene, quality control and record keeping.

Britain and Ireland tend to be conservative in terms of the tradition of prescribing herbal remedies, whereas in France, for example, the medical profession has listed forty medical conditions for which something in the region of 137 plants can be used. Germany is even more advanced in the sense that it permits a much broader range of herbal medicines than anywhere else. Gradually, however, conservative attitudes are changing here. I believe much of the historical reticence on the part of the medical profession is born out of concern for patient welfare and proper standards, and not because of any wish to usurp the role of alternative therapy practitioners, or worries about ceding power and control to them. Patient/consumer protection and quality control remain the key issues.

Bit by bit, attitudes are changing. The recent introduction of degree courses in herbal medicine in two British universities is a reflection of that change.

The Medical Herbalist's Approach

According to the National Institute of Medical Herbalists, the oldest body of its kind in the world, herbalism is the most widely practised form of medicine, with over eighty per cent of the world's population relying on herbs for health. If you are considering using such a herbalist, the Institute can help with lists of qualified practitioners in your area; see Useful Addresses, page 104, for contact details.

Medical herbalists are trained to take a holistic approach to illness. In other words, once they have identified the *underlying* cause of a problem, *that*, rather than the symptoms, is what they treat.

Herbal Medicine and Sleep Disorders

Herbal medicine can treat almost any condition patients might take to their doctor. Clearly, this includes sleep problems, of which insomnia is the most common.

Given that most insomnia is lifestyle/stress- rather than diet-related, the Institute claims an excellent success rate in patients who use herbal remedies as a kind of bridge to prepare physically and mentally for the challenge of facing (and hopefully fixing) their lifestyle problems.

Herbal remedies work by relaxing and supporting the nervous system. The main treatments in order of popularity are:

◆ tinctures (as prescribed by a herbalist)
◆ teas (can be bought over the counter by the public)
◆ herbal baths.

Tinctures

Tinctures are extracts of herbs in a water and alcohol base. Not all herbal tinctures are made up exactly the same. Differences are dictated by a combination of the patient's presenting symptoms and the herbalist's professional judgment. A typical herbalist's remedy for insomnia may contain some or all of the following: valerian, chamomile, skullcap, hops, vervain, passion flower and lime flowers.

Tinctures are usually made up specially by the herbalist, and supplied in a small bottle. The regime is very easy to follow. They are usually taken about three times a day, and in the case of insomnia, a typical course of treatment lasts about a month.

With both tinctures and teas, the patient normally sees an improvement after about ten days.

Teas

Some patients may prefer to opt for herbal teas rather than tinctures, if they have a history of alcohol intolerance or alcoholism. Or they may have religious or ethical problems about taking something with an alcohol constituent.

Like tinctures, teas are usually made up by a herbalist from chopped plants or dried extracts. They are taken once a day, about one hour before bedtime. A typical insomnia remedy includes a mix of chamomile, valerian and hops. The usual quantity is a heaped teaspoon, which is brewed like a normal tea. Best practice is to use a specially dedicated tea pot and leave the mix to infuse for five to ten minutes.

A word about hops...

Generally, hops are contra-indicated for those suffering from depression; people with nervous/anxiety disorders may be quite depressed without knowing it. Insomnia patients with a history of depression should advise their medical herbalist accordingly. Avoiding hops pillows may also be recommended.

And about caffeine ...

Don't expect herbal remedies to work if drinking lots of tea and coffee is part of your daily regime. The advice for insomnia sufferers is to restrict coffee to mornings only, as it is a very strong stimulant. Reduced consumption of tea is also recommended. Tea also contains caffeine, although it is not as strong as coffee. Alternatives in the form of herbal teas are widely available in supermarkets, health food stores and pharmacies.

Dr Corrigan stresses the importance of checking that the ingredients lists of herbal teas don't include other caffeine-containing herbs such as guarana, mate and cola. Unfortunately, herbal tea labels don't always specify this.

Herbal Baths

Herbal bath remedies are best suited to someone looking for relaxation. They are not designed to treat long-term insomnia.

In a typical regime, a combination of either bath and tincture, or bath and tea might be used, but *never* a combination of all three. This would be considered overload.

A typical mix would comprise a dessertspoon of valerian and hops, wrapped in a muslin or loose weave cloth. A twice weekly regime is the optimum. More frequently is not recommended.

A Typical Course of Treatment

A typical course of treatment with a medical herbalist consists of two or more visits, about two weeks apart.

During the first one, the focus will be primarily on taking a detailed medical history. The detail covers diet and exercise regimes, smoking, alcohol consumption, work, family, relationships — all designed to elicit what helps or hinders the insomnia problem. Diet doesn't usually have a large role to play in insomnia, but advice and counselling are given where bad diet — or vitamin deficiency due to poor diet — is aggravating the problem. This can be particularly relevant where people are extremely stressed and eating badly, consuming too much tea or coffee, or chocolate.

Supplies

The vast majority of herbalists source their products from herbal apothecaries/suppliers, although a proportion may grow and prepare them themselves. Most health food shops have a good supply of herbal teas and drops. At the time of writing, the trend seems to be that shop-bought prepared mixes are more expensive than the equivalent remedies made up by herbalists.

How to Find the Best Practitioner

The National Institute of Medical Herbalists in the UK keeps a register of members in the UK, Scotland as well as Ireland, north and south. Members have the letters MNIMH or FNIMH after their name and have undergone a rigorous four-year training period. See page 106 for the Institute's address and telephone number.

Helen McCormack, a Dublin-based qualified medical herbalist, who deals with all types of conditions, reports good success treating those who have consulted her for help with sleeping problems. Whereas feelings of improvement came fairly quickly for these particular patients, she stresses the importance of not regarding any remedy, herbal or otherwise as a cure-all.

Those will only work temporarily if the fundamental lifestyle/psychological issues are addressed at the same time. Issues might include diet-related activities such as over-consumption of caffeine, chocolate, alcohol, nicotine, or foods high in additives. Psychological issues such as tension, anxiety and stress; lifestyle issues such as lack of exercise, or strenuous exercise late at night; watching over-stimulating television programmes late at night — all are important in relation to disturbed sleep. The appropriate adjustments if doing shift work, as recommended on pages 29–31, also need to be made.

Case Studies

Herbal medicine worked for the following patients. To ensure confidentiality, their names have been changed.

Case Study 1
John

Thirty-year-old John is a fit and otherwise healthy factory worker. He had a very disturbed sleep pattern as a result of working shifts over a period of several years. He tended to have at least one disturbed night a week, as his work rotas varied between 6 a.m. to 2 p.m. and 2 to 10 p.m.

Almost out of the blue, the problem of getting to sleep — or staying asleep — got worse over a period of two months. It reached a crisis point, when John found himself managing only two or three hours' sleep a night. As a result, he felt very tired and starting drinking a few pints of beer each evening, in the hope that would help. Finally, in desperation, he went to his GP for treatment and was prescribed sleeping tablets. As he wasn't too happy about that, John only took them as a last resort.

Finally, a friend then recommended medical herbalist Helen McCormack, who prescribed a sleep mixture of equal parts valerian, skullcap and passion flower, which he took afternoon and evening. She also prescribed a restorative and tonic, in the form of a mixture of oats, St John's wort, vervain, dandelion root and damiana (one teaspoon taken mornings).

On his follow-up visit two weeks later, John claimed that his sleep pattern was immediately restored. He also reported a vast improvement in both energy levels and mood. One year on, he is still well. He takes more exercise and drinks less tea, but otherwise has not made major lifestyle changes.

Case Study 2
Anne

Anne is a forty-six-year-old, full-time home maker, with a recent history of depressive illness, characterised by feeling anxious. She complained of low energy levels, combined with a desire to withdraw from social contact. Anne had been taking Prozac for two years, but felt that while it helped with her anxiety, it made her lethargic.

For a period of several months before consulting Helen McCormack, Anne reported waking up very early and being unable to get back to sleep. During the day, she fretted a lot and, generally, let small problems and issues overtake her. She did not take formal physical exercise, and had stopped attending adult education classes — something she had previously enjoyed a great deal. Her self-esteem was very low, and she was gradually withdrawing from people to the extent that social interaction was by now almost non-existent.

Helen McCormack prescribed a tincture remedy containing equal parts of valerian, vervain, St John's wort, skullcap and oats. Anne took this three times a day for two months, then twice a day for two months. After a period of four weeks, she reported a gradual improvement with the early morning waking. She also reported feeling more robust mentally, and had recently enrolled for self-development classes. Her eating pattern also improved (something she had been neglecting, which had contributed to making her feel lethargic).

After three months, following some additional adjustments to her remedy, Anne had stopped taking Prozac, reported feelings of well-being, had more energy and was more socially involved. Six months on, she remains well, has a brighter outlook on life and is no longer taking herbal medicine.

Case Study 3
Sally

Sally is a twenty-eight-year-old physiotherapist working in a busy hospital. She sought the help of a medical herbalist because of fatigue combined with a disturbed sleeping pattern. She had a very demanding job, had recently returned from an overseas aid work assignment and was finding it very difficult to adjust to life back home. A recent relationship break-up added to her stress and misery.

She described herself as normally a very energetic person with a great zest for life but, lately, was finding it impossible to display much enthusiasm for anything. Despite a very full work schedule and often working overtime, she was finding it very difficult to get to sleep and was becoming more and more exhausted as a result. She was also experiencing increasing numbers of headaches, and some digestive disturbances combined with burning sensations in her stomach.

Added to her psychological stresses, she was getting very little time to eat and often breakfast was her only meal of the day until late in the evening. She took little or no formal exercise. Obviously, these were critical contributory factors to her condition.

Sally's prescription remedy comprised two tinctures of nervines and digestive remedies designed to help her relax more. Chamomile — for digestive problems — was combined with liquorice root and borage — for adrenal gland support — as well as skullcap and vervain for the nervous system. Helen also asked her to get some form of exercise every day and to consider taking yoga if at all possible.

Overall, the treatment programme lasted three months. However, on only her second follow-up visit, Sally reported feeling more relaxed. She had begun to sleep better, had no headaches and was experiencing less digestive disturbances. Although work was still stressful, she was taking time to eat and was walking to work. It was a number of months before she felt fully in control of her life again, but taking herbal remedies coupled with lifestyle changes helped to resolve her problems.

Aromatherapy

Aromatherapy is, arguably, one of the great misnomers — essential oil therapy would probably be a better name. As far as the general public is concerned, it is possibly one of the least understood, yet one of the most beneficial, of the complementary therapies. Enthusiastic practitioners maintain that with regular use of essential oils, they stay healthier, manage to cut down consumption of antibiotics and other medications, and limit their reasons for visits to doctors to only the most serious complaints.

Background

One difficulty is that aromatherapy suffers from an image problem. The word aromatherapy is overused by the cosmetic and bath products industry. It is too closely associated with skin and relaxation therapies, to the detriment of its more serious applications. Essential oil labelling can be inconsistent to say the least. In addition, the number, range and duration of training courses is extensive.

The practice of aromatherapy differs slightly from country to country. For example, where aromatherapy has originated from the UK, massage is an integral part of the training process. In France, however, from where aromatherapy came to the UK, it is a branch of medicine used by medical doctors, who have completed a four-year course on phytotherapy. This includes any therapy using plant material, and massage plays no part in the training. It concentrates on medicinal applications — ingestion, inhalations, compresses, plus forms of intensive use.

Some French beauty therapists use essential oils, but formal training is limited to studying the properties and effects of the oils. They are already qualified in body and/or facial massage, therefore massage techniques may be used by them also.

There are not many scientific studies demonstrating the effectiveness of essential oils in tackling a variety of medical ailments, but there are some. These include studies carried out in Australia, America, Germany and France, verifying anti-bacterial and anti-viral properties of some oils. Other studies have been done in Japan, on the use of peppermint to enhance memory in examinations. More recently, some interesting studies have been carried out on the use of essential oils in hospitals as a possible alternative to sleeping pills, and as a way of reducing stress for patients in intensive care.

Generally, however, the profession suffers from a lack of scientific studies to verify the impressive range of ailments it can help. This is a great pity. There is much empirical evidence about the usefulness of aromatherapy, and proof of its popularity and efficacy lies in the number of referrals aromatherapists receive from happy clients.

How Treatment Works

Pure essential oils are highly penetrative, and can reach the small blood capillaries in the skin within minutes. Reaching the various organs is a different matter. This may take thirty minutes in some people, or several hours in others. It also depends to a certain extent on the essential oil itself. This delay factor is one of the reasons why, after an aromatherapy massage, the oil should not be washed off. A bath or shower should be delayed for at least three to four hours after treatment, to allow for maximum penetration and effectiveness.

Massage is not, of course, the only way to get essential oils into the bloodstream.

Full body massage is the method most often used by the professional aromatherapist, although this is not a prerequisite for successful treatment. Aromatherapy may also involve applications to oneself (preferably using a lotion base); or it may involve inhalations, baths, compresses, gargling or mouth-washes. They can be taken orally (in teas), provided this is done with knowledge.

Because they are so powerful, only minuscule amounts are used. Properly handled, essential oils are not dangerous. The intervention of a qualified practitioner isn't *always* necessary, but it is recommended in certain cases. Buying oils in a pharmacy or retail outlet with trained aromatherapy personnel is also recommended, as a lot of labelling is inadequate or vague.

It is possible to make up home treatments using the instructions set out in books, provided attention is paid to quantities used, and guidelines on the avoidance of certain oils in early pregnancy are respected.

Shirley Price runs an international aromatherapy training school in the UK; she has been practising aromatherapy for over twenty years and is the author of six books on the subject. She says:

It is not easy to define the action of essential oils. When a pharmaceutical company produces a drug, it is designed to attack one thing — sleep, headache, pain, infection, what-ever. With aromatherapy, however, you have a scatter gun effect — one essential oil can affect many different organs or conditions, and that is one of the aspects doctors find difficult to accept. They are used to drugs honing in on particular problems.

Aromatherapy and Sleep Disorders

One of the attractive aspects of aromatherapy from an insomnia sufferer's point of view is that essential oils have no side effects (provided they are used correctly). This is one reason why they are often preferred to medication. Cost is another — they are less expensive than most sleeping pills.

According to Shirley Price:

> In the context of sleep problems, some essential oils help the actual insomnia problem, while at the same time reducing stress, lifting depression, easing respiratory or muscular problems. Essential oils can also alleviate a number of other disorders, like bronchitis, arthritis, or urinary problems, which may be causing the sleeplessness in the first place. This, of course, depends on the oils chosen.

Essential oils can help the process of coming off sleeping pills and tranquillisers, but it is important to get your GP's permission first. Going cold turkey is not a good idea. When combined with aromatherapy, weaning off should not take longer than one to three months.

Aromatherapy is highly individualised. People may have completely different reactions to the same oil, and experimenting with different combinations may be necessary. All essential oils are potent, and should be treated with respect. But be adventurous — don't restrict yourself to just one. Oils are synergistic, and benefits tend to increase when two or more oils are judiciously chosen and used together.

For common sleeping problems like insomnia, juniper, lavender and sweet marjoram are a good choice. Treatments aren't always straightforward, though. Used with care, sometimes a combination of aromatherapy, reflexology or another therapy might be necessary. To an extent it can be a case of trial and error.

The Practitioner's Perspective

Susan Bradshaw, Roisin Moloney and Bernie Redden all worked as nurses for sixteen years before taking an eighteen-month course in aromatherapy, which qualified them to be members of the International Society of Professional Aromatherapists.

They say that aromatherapy is neither a quick-fix solution for someone suffering from medical problems, nor a treatment for life — it falls somewhere in between. They add that not only can it be used to treat and control illness effectively, but, perhaps even more importantly, aromatherapy can help prevent the loss of good health in the first place:

The psychological effects of aromatherapy with massage can be extremely strong. Occasionally, people's emotions can be released with a combination of essential oils and massage. We would advise anyone seeking this treatment to make sure that the aromatherapist has the requisite qualifications, perhaps even including some counselling skills; that the practice carries proper insurance and that the treatment room is precisely that — a private room where the client can release emotions in privacy. We would not favour screened cubicles, as privacy and comfort cannot be guaranteed.

We treat everyone from severely mentally handicapped adults with aggressive personality disorders to mothers and babies with colic, and those suffering with arthritis. The vast majority of clients, however, would probably be those suffering from problems derived from stress, anxiety or bereavement. Sleeping difficulties are extremely common. For those clients, we recommend one treatment a week for six weeks, if they are in an acute or particularly disturbed sleeping pattern. After that, it can be reduced to once every three weeks, continuing for as long as they feel the need/benefit.

Clients with sleeping problems usually attend late afternoon or early evening because the treatment prepares them for sleep, as it were. A full body massage takes about two hours, neck and shoulders about forty-five minutes. The treatment is very powerful. Many people feel so relaxed or light-headed that they cannot trust themselves to drive home, and arrange to be collected.

In between treatments, we advise them to use essential oils in a burner at home (for about forty-five minutes in the bedroom before going to bed), or a total of six to eight drops of different essential oils added to a warm bath — say, lavender, Roman chamomile and sweet marjoram.

Pregnancy is one area where the aromatherapist's advice on the use of essential oils needs to be followed carefully. Cancer is another. There we follow very specific guidelines.

They note that it is important for any therapist to take a detailed medical history. They also make follow-up phone calls to see how their clients are feeling, particularly after a first session.

Case Studies

To see some of the benefits of aromatherapy treatments in practice, two case studies are outlined below. To ensure confidentiality, the names of the people featured have been changed.

Case Study 1
Alice

Thirty-four-year-old Alice is a secretary with a four-year-old son. She developed chronic sleep problems for the first time in her life after her husband died of cancer. (She had spent the previous year nursing him at home.) After her husband's death, Alice attended a bereavement counsellor, who finally recommended aromatherapy. Alice was having terrible difficulty sleeping and coping with her grief — a situation which had continued without improvement for over twelve months.

The aromatherapist's treatment comprised a full body massage, using lavender, sweet marjoram, neroli and rosewood once a week for three weeks. After two weeks, there was a noticeable improvement in Alice's sleep pattern. She slept for longer every night, and stopped waking up with crying fits and nightmares. After ten weeks, her oils were changed to a mixture of lavender, neroli and rose otto.

Two years on, she attends once a month for a full body massage; she is still sleeping well, and looks and feels very well. She has never had to resort to sleeping pills, although a combination of these and aromatherapy would not be contra-indicated. Today, the main benefit Alice derives from aromatherapy is relaxation.

Case Study 2
David

David is thirty-nine years old and at the time he started treatment, he was working as a senior manager in a computer company. He had an extremely stressful job, combined with a highly charged and complicated emotional as well as domestic life. He was referred to Susan Bradshaw in a state of absolute exhaustion, with appalling sleep disturbance — waking every night at 4 a.m. and unable to get back to sleep; feeling wiped out the next day.

David was attending a psychotherapist at the same time, and over a three-month period came once a week for a two-hour full body aromatherapy massage of lavender, sweet marjoram, neroli and rosewood. After five weeks of treatment, his sleep increased from four to six hours. After ten weeks, the oil mix was changed to lavender, marjoram, juniper and sandalwood. At this stage, he took a general look at his life and made some major work and living changes.

The whole treatment period lasted fifteen months, and two years on, David still has no sleep or anxiety problems. He says he feels great, and is glad to have opted for the no-drugs route, combined with aromatherapy and psychological support.

Useful Addresses

Ireland

Autogenic Training
The Priory Clinic, 18 Priory Hall, Stillorgan, Co. Dublin.
Tel. 01 283 5566.

Aware — Helping to Defeat Depression
147 Phibsborough Road, Dublin 7. Tel. 01 830 8449;
Help line 01 679 1711.

Dublin County Stress Clinic
St John of God Hospital, Stillorgan, Co. Dublin.
Tel. 01 288 1781.

Irish Association of Medical Herbalists
186 Philipsburgh Avenue, Marino, Dublin 3. Tel. 01 836 7859.

Irish Medical Acupuncture Society
70 Ranelagh Village, Dublin 6. Tel. 01 660 4810.

Irish Medical Homeopathic Association
115 Morehampton Road, Donnybrook, Dublin 4.
Tel. 01 269 7768.

Irish Narcolepsy Support Group (North/South)
11 Grange Terrace, Blackrock, Co. Dublin. Tel. 01 289 5356.

Irish Yoga Association
108 Lower Kimmage Road, Harold's Cross, Dublin 6.
Tel. 01 492 9213.

Sleep Apnoea Clinic
St Vincent's Hospital, Elm Park, Dublin 4. Tel. 01 269 4533.

The Sleep Disorders Clinic
Mater Private Hospital, 71 Eccles Street, Dublin 7.
Tel. 01 860 0090.

United Kingdom

AOC (Aromatherapy Organisations Council)
3 Latymer Close, Braybrooke, Market Harborough, Leicester
LE16 8LN. Tel. 01858 434242.

Aware — Helping to Defeat Depression
22 Great James's Street, Derry. Tel. 01504 260602.

British Association for Autogenic Training and Therapy
c/o The Royal London Homeopathic Hospital, Great Ormond
Street, London WC1N 3HR.
Note: Postal enquiries only. Please send a stamped addressed
envelope for an information leaflet and a list of registered,
qualified trainers.

British Psychological Society
St Andrew's House, 48 Princess Road East, Leicester
LE1 7DR. Tel. 0116 254 9568.

British Snoring and Sleep Apnoea Association
How Lane, Chipstead, Surrey CR5 3LT. Tel. 01737 557997.

British Sleep Society

PO Box 144, Wakefield, Yorkshire WF4 2XY.

Tel. 01226 380287.

GPs can contact the Society for information on sleep clinics.

British Wheel of Yoga

BWY Central Office, 1 Hamilton Place, Boston Road,
Sleaford, Lincolnshire NG34 7ES. Tel. 01529 306851.

Centre for Stress Management

156 Westcombe Hill, Blackheath, London SE3 7DH.
Tel. 0181 293 4114.

Faculty of Homeopathy

The Royal London Homeopathic Hospital, Great Ormond
Street, London WC1N 3HR. Tel. 0171 837 9469.

Institute of Complementary Medicine

PO Box 194, London SE16 1QZ. Tel. 0171 237 5165.

International Society of Professional Aromatherapists

ISPA House, 82 Ashby Road, Hinckley, Leicestershire
LE10 1SN. Tel. 01455 637987.

Manic Depression Fellowship

8 High Street, Kingston upon Thames, Surrey KT1 1EY.
Tel. 0181 974 6550.

National Institute of Medical Herbalists

56 Longbrook Street, Exeter EX4 6AH. Tel. 01392 426022.

Oxford Sleep Unit

Osler Chest Unit, Churchill Hospital, Headington, Oxford
OX3 7LJ. Tel. 01865 225236.

Sleep

Respiratory Support and Sleep Centre
Papworth Hospital, Papworth Everard, Cambridge CB3 8RE.
Tel. 01480 830541.

SANELINE
199 Old Marylebone Road, London NW1 5QP.
Tel. 0171 724 8000; 0345 678000.

Shirley Price Aromatherapy
Essentia House, Upper Bond Street, Hinckley, Leicestershire
LE10 1RS. Tel. 01455 615466.

Sleep Apnoea Trust
Warwick Lodge, Piddington Lane, Piddington, High Wycombe,
Buckinghamshire HP14 3BD. Tel. 01494 838778.

Sleep Assessment and Advisory Service
PO Box 21, Lisburn, Co. Antrim BT28 2SF. Tel. 01846 622266.

Sleep Disorders Centre
The Lane-Fox Unit, St Thomas's Hospital, Lambeth Palace
Road, London SE1 7EH. Tel. 0171 928 9292.

Sleep Disorders Clinic
Neurosciences Unit, King's Healthcare, Denmark Hill,
London SE5. Tel. 0171 919 3407.

Sleep Matters Self-Help Group (Insomnia)
PO Box 3087, London W4 4ZP. Tel. 0181 994 9874.

Sleep Laboratory, Edinburgh Royal Infirmary
Lauriston Place, Edinburgh EH3 9YW. Tel. 0131 536 1000.

UK Narcolepsy Association
1 Brook Street, Stoke on Trent ST4 1JN. Tel. 01782 416417.

Further Reading

Benson, Herbert and Miriam Z. Klipper, *Relaxation Response*, New York: Avon Books 1976.

Berridge, John, C.L. Cooper and C. Highley, *Employee Assistance Programmes and Workplace Counselling*, New York: John Wiley & Sons Inc. 1997.

Borysenko, Joan, *Minding the Body, Mending the Mind*, New Jersey: Bantam Press 1993.

Boyne, Edward (ed.), *A Guide to Psychotherapy in Ireland*, Dublin: Columba Press 1993.

Burns, David D., *Feeling Good Handbook: Using the New Mood Therapy in Everyday Life*, Victoria: Plume Books 1989.

Burton, Tim and Steve Palmer, *Dealing with People Problems at Work*, McGraw 1995.

Cooper, Cary L. and Sue Cartwright, *Managing Workplace Stress*, London: Sage Publications 1997.

Corrigan, Desmond, *Herbal Medicine for Sleep and Relaxation*, UK: Amberwood Publishing 1996.

Covey, Stephen R., *Seven Habits of Highly Effective People: Powerful Lessons in Personal Change*, New Jersey: Simon & Schuster 1992.

Hayden, Fionnuala, *Whose Housework Is It Anyway?*, Dublin: Marino Press 1995.

Hopson, Barrie and Mike Scally, *Time Management: Conquer the Clock*, Mercury Business Books 1996.

Keane, Colm (ed.), *The Stress File*, Dublin: Blackwater Press 1997.

Keane, Colm, *Nervous Breakdown*, Dublin: Mercier Press 1994.

Kenton, Leslie, *10 Day De-stress Plan: Make Stress Work for You*, London: Ebury Press 1994.

Kenton, Susannah and Leslie Kenton, *Endless Energy: A Workbook for Dynamic Health and Personal Power for Women on the Move*, London: Vermilion 1993.

Kermani, Kai, *Autogenic Training: Effective Holistic Way to Better Health*, London: Souvenir Press 1996.

Lockie, Andrew, *The Family Guide to Homeopathy*, London: Hamish Hamilton.

Palmer, Stephen and Lynda Strickland, *Stress Management: A Quick Guide*, Cambridge: Daniels Medica 1995.

Peale, Norman Vincent, *Power of Positive Thinking*, UK: Mandarin 1990.

Price, Shirley, *Aromatherapy for Common Ailments*, London: Gaia Books 1991.

Scott, Elizabeth, *The Natural Way to Sound Sleep*, London: Orion Books 1996.

Weekes, Claire, *Self Help for Your Nerves*, London: Thorsons 1995.

Weil, Andrew, *Eight Weeks to Optimum Health*, London: Warner 1997.

Index

actigraphy, 14

acupuncture, 83–5

adolescents, 11

age, 7

alcohol, 2, 19–20, 39–40, 48

   jet lag, 24

   sleep apnoea, 34

allergies, 20, 45

American Sleep Disorders Association, 36

anaemia, 22

anorexia nervosa, 43

anti-depressants, 36, 55, 57–61, 82

   recommendations, 61–3

anxiolytic drugs, 59

aromatherapy, 42, 44, 97–103

   case studies, 102–3

asthma, 20, 45, 46

autogenic training, 74–9

   process of, 77–9

   and sleep disorders, 76–7

barbiturates, 58

bathing, 42, 49, 92

bedroom, 45–7

benzodiazepines, 58–9, 88–9

beta-blockers, 21

Bhagavad Gita, 50

Bhopal leak, 5

blood pressure, 21

blood sugar, 81

body clock disorders, 16

body temperature, 9

Bradshaw, Susan, 100–102, 103

British Association for Autogenic Training and Therapy (BAFATT), 75

British Sleep Society, 9

bruxism, 16, 38

caffeine, 40, 48, 81, 92

cataplexy, 37

Challenger space shuttle, 5

Chan Mullen, Dr Katherine, 83–5

Chernobyl disaster, 5

children

   sleep apnoea, 34

chronotherapy, 72

circadian rhythms, 7–10

   peaks and valleys, 8

complementary medicine, 86–103

continuous positive airway pressure (CPAP), 35, 70–71

core sleep, 6–7

Corrigan, Dr Desmond, 87–9

cot death, 34

counselling, 57

Crowe, Dr Catherine, 6, 22, 28–9

   clinical treatment, 67, 68, 71, 72

day-time sleepiness, 37

depression, 13, 42, 76

case studies, 63–7

checklist, 62–3

effects on sleep, 16, 18, 56

symptoms, 3, 61–3

Dexedrine, 37

diabetes, 20, 22, 76

diet, 41, 47–8

shift work, 30

digestion, 8–9

disturbed sleep, vii–viii

diuretics, 20, 21

doctors, 55–7

use of drugs, 59–61

drugs, 37, 40, 55–61

case studies, 63–7

doctor's dilemma, 59–61

Edison, Thomas, 4

endocrine diseases, 20

essential oils, 44–5, 97–103

European Sleep Research Society, 6

exercise, 30, 41, 48–9

Fitzpatrick, Dr Brendan, 80–82

food. see diet

foot bath, 42–3

frequency, 20, 48

geranium, 45

Gleadhill, Dr Iain, 31–2

Greene, Dr Alice, 74–5, 77–9

heart disease, 21

herbal remedies, 30, 42, 87–97

baths, 90, 92

case studies, 94–7

course of treatment, 92–3

teas, 91

tinctures, 90, 91

homeopathy, 79–83

and sleep disorders, 82–3

hops, 42, 89

hypersomnia, 16

hypnogogic hallucinations, 37

hypnotic drugs, 58–61

hypoglycaemia, 20

Idzikowski, Dr Chris, vii–viii, 9, 11, 17

insomnia, 15, 16, 17–21

aggravating factors, 19–21

among older people, 17–18, 21–3

definition of, 18–19

investigation of, 69

International Society of Professional Aromatherapists, 100

ioniser, 46

jet lag, 23–8

medications, 27–8

reducing effects of, 24–7

lavender, 42, 44

light therapy, 30–31, 72–3

Lindemann, Dr Hannes, 75

McCormack, Helen, 93–5

mandarin, 45

massage, 43, 98–9

melatonin, 17–18, 27

menopause, 20, 21, 42, 51

microsleep, 5

mid-afternoon dip, 8

Moloney, Roisin, 100–102

multiple sleep latency test, 69

Murray, Dr Tiernan, 56–7, 58, 61

case studies, 63–7

naps, 10, 12, 43, 69

narcolepsy, 13, 36–8

National Institute of Medical
  Herbalists, 90, 93
neroli, 45
nicotine, 29, 46–7
night owl syndrome, 72
night shift. *see* shift work
night terrors, 16
NREM sleep, 6–7

oils, 44–5
orthopaedic mattress, 46

pets, 45
phytotherapy, 97
pillows, 46
polysomnography, 68–70
Price, Shirley, 99, 100
problems, 12–13
psycho-active drugs, 58–9

Redden, Bernie, 100–102
regular hours, 40–41
relaxation tape, 42
REM related phenomena, 37
REM sleep, 3, 6–7, 9
renal failure, 22
restless legs syndrome, 16, 22–3,
  81
Ritalin, 37
road traffic accidents, 2, 3, 5
Roman chamomile, 45
room temperature, 41, 45–6

sandalwood, 45
shift work, 17, 20, 28–31
  do's and don'ts, 29–31
skin disorders, 20
sleep
  amount needed, 11–15
  cycles, 1
  disorders of, 16–38
  experiment, 13–14

historical background, 4–5
investigation of, 68–73
necessity of, 5
patterns, 2
stages of, 6–10
sleep apnoea, 13, 16, 31, 32–6
  clinical treatment, 70–71
  diagnosis, 34–5
  investigation of, 69
  sufferers, 33–4
  treatment, 35–6
sleep clinics, 13, 68–73
sleep diary, 13–14
sleep paralysis, 37
sleeping pills, 1, 3, 20, 27, 43
  coming off, 67
  extent of use, 4
  recommendations, 55–61
  shift work, 30
  snoring, 32
sleep-walking, 16
smoking, 2–3, 29, 33, 46–7
snoring, 16, 31–2
Southgate, Linda, 50–51, 53–4
Sudden Infant Death Syndrome,
  34
surgery
  sleep apnoea, 35
sweet marjoram, 44–5

teas, 91
technology, 69–70
teeth grinding, 16, 38
television, 42, 47
Three Mile Island accident, 5
tinctures, 91

urination, frequent, 20, 48

valerian, 1, 30, 88–9
vitamin deficiency, 48

waking at night, 9–10, 14–15

weight, 2, 34

    sleep apnoea, 35, 36

    sleep pattern, 43

World Health Organisation, 17

yoga, 49–52

    case studies, 53–4